# THE DOSE
# MAKES
# THE POISON

## A GUIDE TO FLEXIBLE DIETING

## ACADIA BURO
### ILLUSTRATED BY HANNAH MERCHANT

Copyright © 2018 Acadia Buro and Hannah Merchant.

All rights reserved.

ISBN: 1981969683
ISBN-13: 9781981969685

To our family

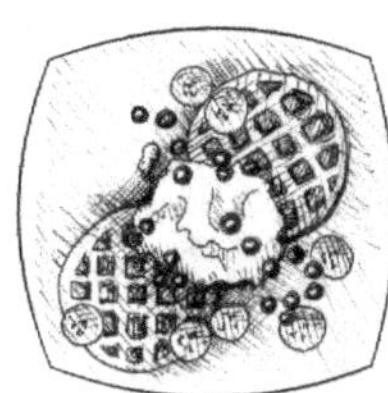

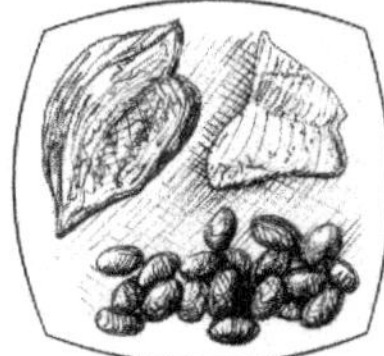

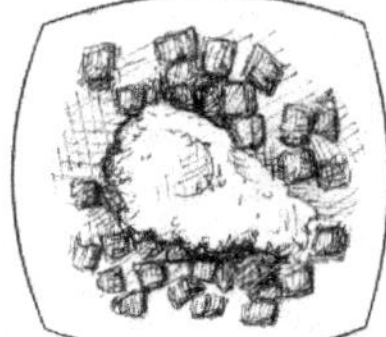

# CONTENTS



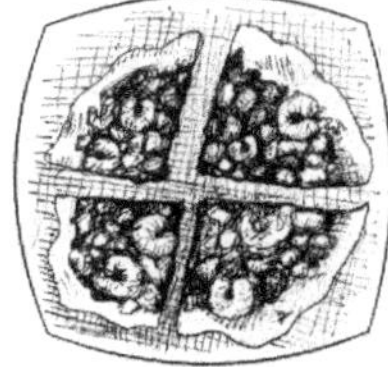

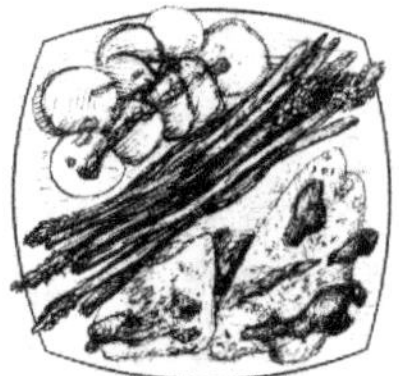

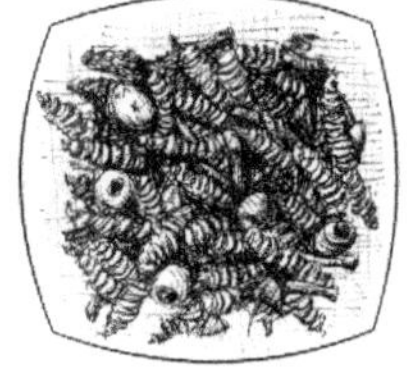

# 1

# INTRODUCTION

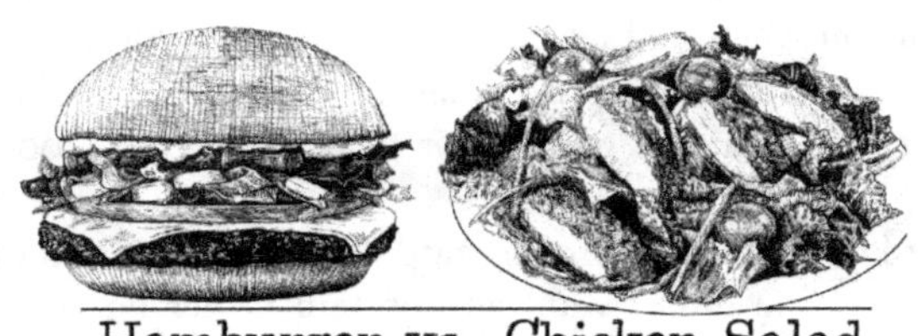



| | | |
|---|---|---|
| CALS | 760 | 1290 |
| FAT | 45g | 85g |
| SAT FAT | 15g | 13g |
| SODIUM | 1140mg | 2300mg |
| CARB | 44g | 84g |
| FIBER | 2g | 11g |
| SUGAR | 7g | 52g |
| PROTEIN | 46g | 51g |

Which is the smarter option? A salad or a burger? The salad has vegetables, and vegetables contain plenty of vitamins and minerals. Leafy greens take up plenty of volume in your stomach to make you feel full and contain fiber to keep you feeling full after the meal is over. The burger has saturated fat and refined, white carbohydrates, which are "bad," right? Plus, I think I remember reading somewhere that red meat is bad for you.

These choices can have more similar nutritional values than you might expect, with the salad often containing more carbohydrates, fat, and overall calories than the burger. Let's look at two menu options from the same chain restaurant.

A hamburger has 760 calories, 45 g of fat (15 g saturated), 1,140 mg sodium, 44 g of carbohydrates (2 g fiber, 7 g sugar), and 41 g of protein. If we add cheese, we are at 52 g fat and 46 g protein. A grilled chicken salad at the same restaurant has 1,290 calories, 85 g fat (13 g saturated), 2,300 mg sodium, 84 g carbohydrates (11 g fiber, 52 g sugar), and 51 g protein.

These are both calorie-dense meals, but with nearly half the fat, carbohydrate, and total calorie content with similar protein content, the burger is the clear winner. Sodium content is much higher for the salad, and the saturated fat content is virtually the same between the two. In any case, you would be better off cooking food at home or asking for substitutions to improve the nutritional profile of your meal than ordering either of these items. When you take away salad dressing and some calorie-dense toppings, the carbohydrate and fat content will decrease. If you skip the cheese and opt for grilled chicken or ahi tuna instead of a ground-beef burger, you can watch the fat content of the meal plummet as well. All that is required to be successful with your diet is an understanding of how much you need to be eating to reach your goals and which foods will get you there.

Yesterday at Chipotle I overheard the woman in front of me explain to her friend that she didn't want any protein in her bowl because she was watching her weight. Here is what she ordered: a hearty portion of white rice, fajita vegetables, mild salsa, sour cream, and lettuce. She explained to her friend that cheese and guacamole were both high in fat, which is why she did not order either. Based on my observations, I am guessing that this woman is following a low-fat, low-protein diet and that she doesn't know sour cream is high in fat. I don't know what else she ate that day, so I can't say whether she is trying to count calories or not.

For fear of being rude, I kept my mouth shut, but here is what I wanted to say: protein is the most satiating macronutrient. Without the addition of a protein source, your bowl would have made your blood sugar and insulin levels spike and left you feeling hungry soon after you finished it were it not for the huge blob of sour cream, which contains more fat than the cheese you avoided ordering due to its high fat content. In fact, 9 of the 13 g of total fat and 7 of the 7.5 g of saturated fat in her meal came from the sour cream.

Based on Chipotle's nutrition calculator, her order contained 370 calories, making it a very low-calorie meal. However, the portions measured out by the employees (despite great effort on their part) rarely match the portions used in their published nutrition data. The customer did not ask them to go light on the rice or sour cream, and I could tell the portions were much larger than what would yield a 370-calorie meal. Again, I don't know what else she ate that day, so she could very well be on track to losing weight and reaching her goals.

However, what struck me was not her meal itself but rather her apparent lack of knowledge about the three macronutrients. Chipotle's calculator also tells me that her order contained 13 g of fat, 49 g of carbohydrates, and 7 g of protein. Again, her actual meal likely contained much more food than what the calculator describes. If her other meals are higher in protein and her overall caloric intake is below what she needs to maintain her weight, she is on track. Based on my observations of her conduct, my educated guess is that her other meals do not meet both requirements, in which case she requires more knowledge to be able to achieve her goals. Protein is not magic, but it is the most satiating macronutrient. For that reason, calorie-restricted, high-protein diets are extremely effective. Of course, there are other simple tools to optimize progress that we will discuss later.

You may have heard about someone losing weight by eating at Chipotle every day. I myself have done this. You may have heard of someone eating ice cream, pizza, or even at McDonald's every day and losing weight. In fact, it is entirely possible to meet your physique and health goals while doing any of the above. How? Flexible dieting is the answer.

"Flexible dieting," sometimes used interchangeably with "If It Fits Your Macros" (IIFYM), describes a way of eating that involves tracking not only your caloric intake but also the nutrient composition of your diet. The term "flexible" refers to the fact that you can be flexible about how you reach your calorie and nutrient goals as long as you reach them. Similarly, the term "IIFYM" comes from the notion that you can eat whatever you want if it "fits" in your macronutrient goals. While the two terms are sometimes used to describe the same approach, in this book, flexible dieting refers to an approach that is more personalized and more balanced than IIFYM. Flexible dieting combines scientific evidence with your individual wants and needs to create a nutritional approach that is most appropriate and effective for you.

Many successful diets rely on calorie counting. Calorie restriction is in fact the key to weight loss, just as caloric excess is the key to weight gain. For anyone interested in more specific goals related to body composition, athletic performance, or overall health, paying attention to specific nutrients in addition to calories is essential. This is exactly what flexible dieting does. Flexible dieting takes mindful eating one layer deeper than calorie counting to consider the various nutrients that make up our food. Calorie counting tells us how much to eat; nutrient tracking helps guide us toward what to eat. Many flexible dieters ignore calories when tracking their intake and stick only to macronutrients. In theory, the math works out the same; it is simply easier to track three numbers (macronutrients) than four (macronutrients and calories).

Attention to both quantity and quality is required to reach nutrition-related goals. Without guidance on both how much and what types of food to eat, our approach to dieting will always be less than optimal. For instance, in contrast to the calorie-counting approach lies the "clean eating" camp. Clean eating requires consuming a diet rich in whole foods but says nothing about quantity. If we ignore our macronutrient and calorie requirements, we are left with a different but equally problematic situation to that imposed by simple calorie counting. Of course, people who "eat clean" and track their macronutrient intake can solve this problem. The solution is to account for both quantity and quality in our diets. But what many people do not realize is that if we eat varied diets full of foods from most or all food groups, then diet quality is innately good, and quantity is what we really need to focus on.

I have seen plenty of overweight people fill their diets with nutritious foods and make sure to exercise yet cannot understand why they are not seeing results. What are they doing wrong? First, they might not be measuring portions. Next, they might be trying to make the food taste better by adding more ingredients, which can be a recipe for disaster. Adding large quantities of oil, butter, cheese, or cream to vegetables changes the nutrient composition of the dish entirely. Even though these people are getting adequate nutrients, their healthy eating habits are backfiring because they are consuming too many calories, which can lead not only to weight gain but also to poor metabolic outcomes and potentially an increased risk of disease. The bottom line is that if you eat too much of anything, even if it's the most organic, sugar-free, gluten-free, dairy-free, non-GMO diet in existence, you will still gain weight.

Additionally, those who are measuring portions without paying attention to macronutrients are missing out on a key factor to success. Each of the three macronutrients has different effects on our body. If we compare two sample diets with the same number of calories but different macronutrient ratios, we can see that one would leave us feeling satisfied, energized, and primed to meet our body composition and health goals, while the other would leave us hungry, tired, and unable to effectively meet our goals.

Diet 1

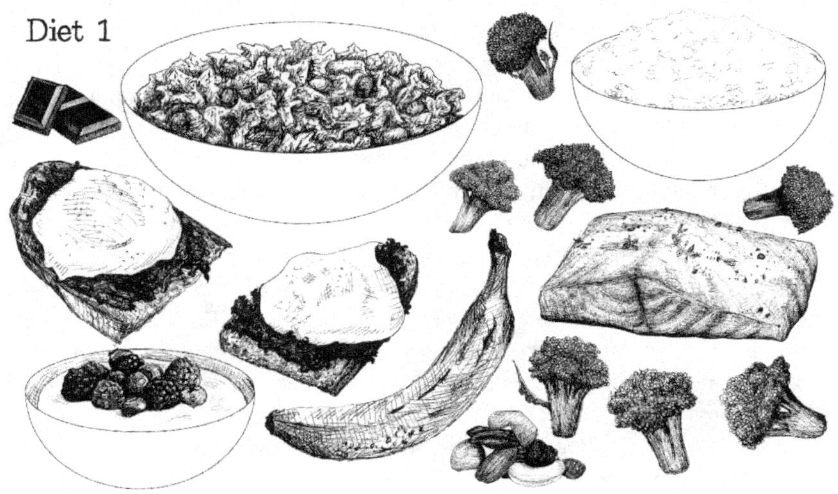

# Comparison of Two Diets
## with Similar Caloric Intake

Diet 2

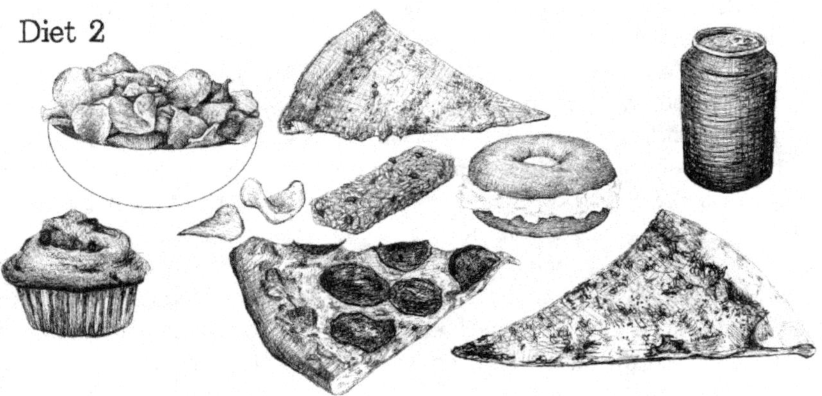

Diet 1: 2 poached eggs on greens on toast, greek yogurt with berries, banana, large salad with beans and chicken, salmon with rice and broccoli, handful of nuts, and a square of chocolate.

Diet 2: bagel with cream cheese, muffin, granola bar, chips, 3 pieces of pizza, soda.

Flexible dieting gained popularity within the bodybuilding community as a method to gain muscle or achieve extremely low levels of body fat while still enjoying one's favorite foods. But the movement is growing, and flexible dieting is a useful tool for anyone looking to simultaneously take care of his or her physical and mental health.

The beauty of flexible dieting is that it allows you to reach specific nutrition-related goals with the option of never having to prepare your own meals. You can diet and retain your social life, your comfort, and let yourself pursue all the wonderful opportunities that life has to offer. How flexible you want to be is truly up to you. You can eat out for every meal or prepare everything yourself. You can eat something different for each meal or repeat the same meal plan every day. You have complete control over the way you reach your health and fitness goals. The only requirement is that the numbers add up correctly.

Unlike many other approaches to dieting, flexible dieting allows you to eat with mindfulness and intention without anyone else ever having to know that you are following a specific diet plan. With flexible dieting, you can literally diet for months without anyone knowing you are on a diet. It is likely that you are the only one who knows what you do 24/7, so you are likely the only one who knows how many total calories you consume and how much total physical activity you perform. For this reason, much of the anecdotal evidence throughout this book comes from my own experiences, since I can say with certainty only what I have experienced.

Unless you have a diagnosis, allergy, or intolerance, a flexible dieting approach does not require that you eliminate anything from your diet. Sugar, gluten, bread, artificial sweeteners, processed foods, carbohydrates, fat, dairy, fruit, soy, red meat, and others are commonly targeted as culprits that will make us gain weight or become unhealthy. But, as we will discuss in the following pages, the culprit is the amount of the food that we consume, and not the food itself.

The phrase "the dose makes the poison" is credited to philosopher and physician Paracelsus, who was born in the fifteenth century. The principle associated with the phrase is that anything can be toxic in excess. Abusing a medication that could save your life if taken in its prescribed dose could kill you. Abusing food that could promote health and well-being if consumed in moderation could contribute to sickness and distress.

The 2015–2020 USDA Dietary Guidelines advise us to follow a healthy eating pattern across a lifespan; to focus on variety, nutrient density, and amount of food; to limit calories from added sugars and saturated fats and reduce sodium intake; to shift to healthier food and beverage choices; and to support healthy eating patterns for all. The guidelines give further recommendations on how to apply these guidelines to your life. The information is available, yet it is not being used by many of us. There is a disconnect between the recommendations and information that exist and the diets that we choose to follow.

This book explains that having your own specific, adaptable, numeric guidelines can be the connection between these abstract guidelines and your personal health and fitness. We can reprogram our decision making about food by establishing rules that must be followed, rules that we must trust more than our own decisions. We are not always logical, reasonable beings. Our internal homeostatic systems are not even always logical. We act impulsively, emotionally. For an exceptional review of our internal hunger regulation systems, refer to Dr. Stephan Guyenet's Hungry Brain: Outsmarting the Instincts That Make Us Overeat.

In this book, I propose that we can override these internal regulation systems by turning instead to external regulation. Tracking your dietary intake to make sure you reach daily calorie, macronutrient, and micronutrient goals can provide this external regulation. In this book, I will discuss ways to optimize success based on scientific data, but more importantly, I will emphasize that an approach that brings you joy will always be the preferred method.

# 2
# WHY FLEXIBLE DIETING WORKS

Flexible dieting encourages you to see your daily calorie requirement as a budget. The total budget is split into three smaller budgets: protein, carbohydrates, and fat. Some of us have a higher spending limit than others based on genetics alone, but our budget can change based on our current lifestyle and goals. For example, just by increasing our physical activity level, we can increase our budget.

When you start flexible dieting, you will learn how to budget your calories so you can save to spend on your favorite foods. You will learn that some foods can fill you up without costing much, while others will leave you hungry for more after you spend a good chunk of your daily total on them. Foods that are nutrient dense will give you the most "bang for your buck." When you spend calories on these foods, you are being thrifty or smart. When you spend calories on foods that are calorie-dense but low in nutrients, it is a splurge.

It is wise to spend most of your budget on sources of lean protein, whole grains, fruit, and vegetables. These can be equated to your bills, savings, and groceries. It can also be fun to save some of your budget for foods like ice cream, pizza, and cookies. These are your new outfits, trips, and event tickets.

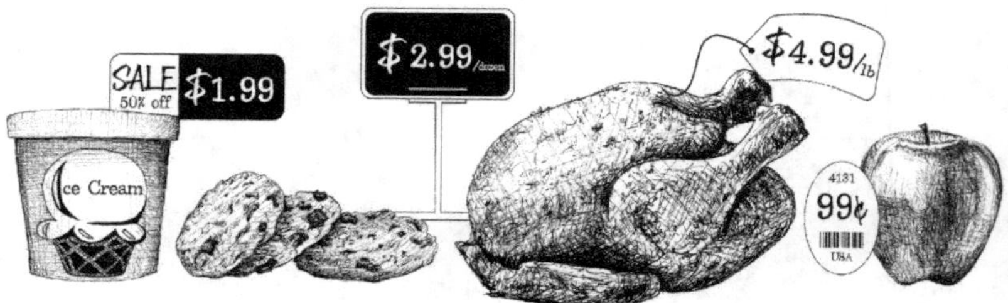


Developing an awareness of your daily calorie and macronutrient budget takes the guesswork out of dieting. Eating for your goals becomes like managing your bank account. Just like with money, once you know your diet budget, it is completely up to you how you manage it.

# Energy Balance

Many diets can work effectively if we stick to them. Low-carb diets, low-fat diets, diets with meal replacement shakes, and diets that force you to eliminate dozens of food choices—they can all work. The reason why these diets work is not that there are secrets to their success but rather that they restrict calories. (Low-carb diets often work without intentional restriction, but because they are so satiating, the overall caloric content often ends up being similar to the caloric content of intentionally calorie-restricted diets.) Any time you are restricting calories, you will lose weight. There are very rare instances where calorie restriction will result in a plateau or weight regain (e.g. in patients after bariatric weight loss surgery). Weight loss is simply about calories ingested versus calories expended.

We derive energy from the food that we eat. In many cases, we measure energy in joules, but when it comes to food, we use an older unit of measure, the calorie. When we talk about calories in food, we are talking about kilocalories, or Calories with an uppercase C. But the generally accepted notation is just "calorie." The relation between the food we consume that inputs calories and the activities we perform that output calories is called energy balance. When either input or output is greater than the other, energy balance tips in one direction, and weight is either lost or gained. Any time we eat or drink, we consume calories. Any time we perform an activity, from digesting food or breathing air to running or weightlifting, we burn calories. When we consume the same amount that we burn, input equals output, so our weight stays the same. If calories consumed exceed calories burned, we gain weight; if calories burned exceed calories consumed, we lose weight.

It is important to note that it is the average of this balance over time that determines whether we maintain, gain, or lose weight. One day of exercise will not make you lose weight. One day of overeating or undereating may or may not tip the scale in either direction depending on other factors like hormones; sodium, water, and fiber intake; when food was last consumed; and how much food was last consumed. Daily fluctuations in weight do not accurately reflect energy balance, but weight over time absolutely does.

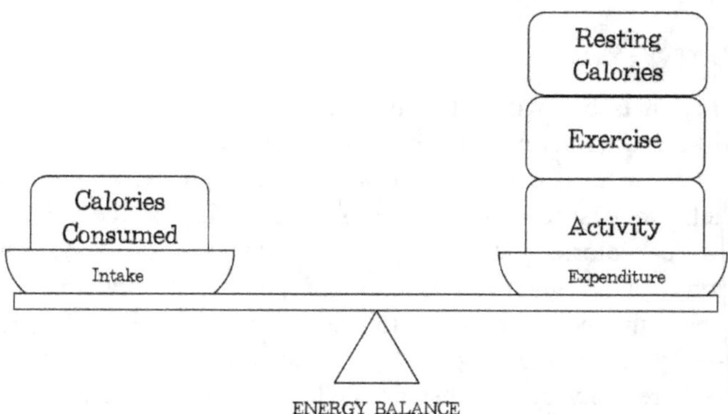


In 2010, Dr. Mark Taub illustrated how energy balance works by losing twenty-seven pounds in two months on a "convenience-store diet" of Hostess and Little Debbie snacks, chips, and sugary cookies and cereals. Many of us would label these foods "bad" or "unhealthy," but because Dr. Taub consumed less calories than he was expending, he lost weight. By losing this weight, he transformed from an overweight to a normal BMI (body mass index, an indicator of whether someone is underweight, normal weight, overweight, or obese), his LDL or "bad" cholesterol decreased, his HDL or "good" cholesterol increased, and his triglyceride levels (fat in the blood) decreased. He was therefore able to reduce risk factors of metabolic diseases by eating "junk food."

Although Dr. Taub lost weight quickly, it is unclear whether he would be able to continue his success on this diet. Each of us has a bodyweight "set point," which is a weight at which we can remain with little or no effort. It turns out that our bodyweight regulation is lopsided in that we have evolved to favor fat storage. The hypothalamus, or part of the brain that regulates temperature, hunger, and thirst, will try to stabilize us back to our set point when we start to drop any weight by increasing hunger and decreasing satiety and by gradually reducing our basal metabolic rate (BMR), which represents the amount of energy expended at rest at room temperature in a post-absorptive state, that is, when your digestive system is not active. Because of the adaptations that occur as we gain or lose weight, successful flexible dieting involves adapting our diet as our body tries to bring us back to our set point. This is especially important when dieting, as our bodies seemingly do everything they can to get us back to our set point. We will discuss more about this in the "Long-Term Success" chapter.

"I don't eat enough" is a common excuse for not losing weight; many believe that if they are not eating enough, then their metabolism will slow down so much that they won't be able to lose any weight. We need to consider an individual's energy balance equation and diet history to find out if they in fact aren't eating "enough." (Hint: usually, they are eating too much.) Is it possible to slow down our metabolism by not eating enough? When someone thinks "not eating enough" is the reason why he or she is having trouble losing weight, the most likely explanation is underestimation of dietary intake. Very often we forget to tally up our snacking or do not realize how calorie-dense meals and drinks are when we go out to eat. It is possible for metabolic rate to decrease if you have been dieting for a very long time or if you are following a very low-calorie diet. In these cases, you may want to take a break from dieting before jumping back in. Rarely, there may be another underlying cause preventing weight loss. You should always check with your doctor or health professional before beginning a diet to make sure there are no major diagnoses or causes for concern. In most cases, however, the problem is that our expectation of energy balance doesn't match reality.

Bodyweight regulation does not occur despite our actions; it occurs because of our actions. In other words, we are not slaves to bodyweight regulation. Just because our internal signals tell us we want to eat calorie-dense foods whenever they are available so that we can store as much body fat as possible does not mean we must listen to these signals. In fact, by making smart choices, we can even override some of these signals.

## Beyond Weight

When we talk about weight, we sometimes ignore the fact that all weight is not the same. Fat mass includes all the fat stores in our body. Lean mass is everything else: organs, bones, water, and muscle. A "healthy" body weight does not guarantee that you are a healthy individual. You can be physically fit and overweight. You can be slim and suffer from or be at risk of metabolic syndrome, a clustering of at least three of five of the following: abdominal obesity, high blood pressure, high fasting blood glucose, high serum triglyceride, and low HDL cholesterol. Unlike weight loss, fat loss depends not only on caloric intake but also nutrient composition of one's diet and duration, intensity, and frequency of physical activity. By combining calorie counting with macronutrient composition, flexible dieting allows you to build a diet with the appropriate portions of each macronutrient for your body that is consistent with your goals.

This is where diets that advocate for "clean eating" or eliminating certain "bad" foods sometimes miss the target. I have seen people make huge lifestyle changes to lose weight but never reach their goals because they didn't adequately measure or even consider their portion sizes. Sure, cutting out bread or eating more vegetables can help you lose weight, but only if it helps you achieve the goal of eating less overall.

To lose fat, you must reduce overall caloric intake, consume enough protein to support muscle maintenance or growth, and follow a resistance training regimen. These steps are critical to minimize weight lost from muscle. Losing fat while preserving muscle will result in what many of us like to call a "toned" look.

Gaining lean mass is similarly complex. A common response to someone trying to gain weight is, "You're so lucky!" Such comments fail to appreciate that gaining healthy weight is a slow, difficult process. To gain a large amount of fat mass quickly, simply remain sedentary and add heavy cream or oil to your diet for some quick, easy, drinkable calories. (Fat has over twice the calories per gram that carbohydrates and protein have.) The surplus will go directly to your fat cells, and voilà! But this is not what we are talking about when we talk about gaining muscle. Gaining lean mass is just as tedious of a process as losing fat. To gain muscle, you need to increase overall caloric intake, consume enough protein to support muscle growth, consume enough carbohydrates and fat to fuel workouts and build muscle, and follow a resistance training regimen.

Alternately, we can spend decades using a flexible dieting approach and end up at the exact same weight at which we started but with improved health markers and body composition. This is sometimes called body recomposition, and it can be a good reminder that weight is just one small tool that we can use to measure the bigger picture of our overall health.

## Understanding Your Diet

Many of us fall into traps thinking we are making "healthy" choices because a meal contains whole foods or is advertised as being loaded with nutrients. Let's consider an example of each. In the first case, we go to a vegan restaurant and order a plate of brown rice, beans, sweet potato, kale, and seasonal vegetables. We may or may not order a meat substitute. It doesn't matter for our example. The meal is cooked in olive oil, a "healthy fat," but the oil is not used sparingly. Depending on the individual, this meal could provide nearly enough carbohydrates or fat to fill an entire day's worth of eating. In another case, let's opt for an acai bowl filled with fruit and granola. The extremely high-calorie, carbohydrate, and simple-sugar contents make this a great option for an endurance athlete preparing for or refueling after a race, but if you are just going to be sitting on the couch all day, it probably is not your best option.

## FOODS WITH THE SAME NUTRIENT CONTENT

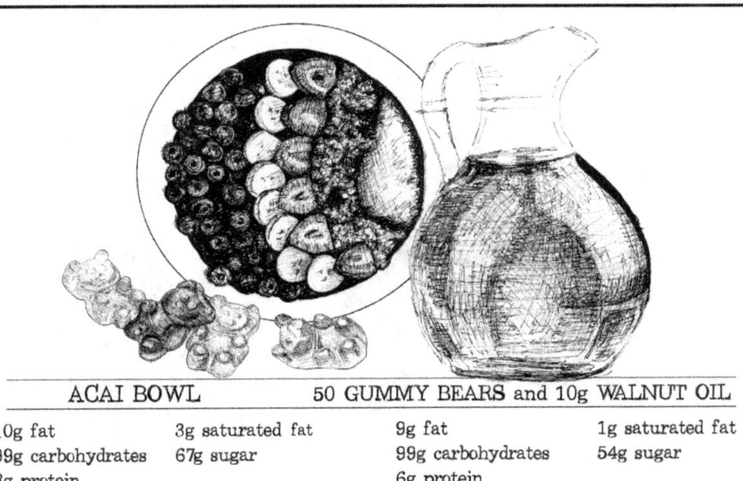

| ACAI BOWL | | 50 GUMMY BEARS and 10g WALNUT OIL | |
|---|---|---|---|
| 10g fat | 3g saturated fat | 9g fat | 1g saturated fat |
| 99g carbohydrates | 67g sugar | 99g carbohydrates | 54g sugar |
| 8g protein | | 6g protein | |

Perhaps the most dangerous of all "health" traps is the salad trap. Salad is supposed to be a safe choice for dieters, but a deli sandwich can sometimes be more diet-friendly. Remember our example from the beginning of this book: the salad versus the burger. Carefully read the toppings and dressings because the fat, sugar, and calories can add up fast.

Most diets that work require an awareness of what you eat, but not all of them require an understanding of how the food you eat will affect you. This is where flexible dieting can take you far beyond the results that you can get on another diet. Flexible dieting requires an understanding of the components that make up our food and the roles that these components play in our bodies. The energy balance equation compares calories ingested to calories expended, but not all calories have the same effect on our body.

In terms of energy, a calorie is a calorie. One calorie always provides the same amount of energy. But in terms of the overall effect on our body, "a calorie is a calorie" is a misleading statement. Macronutrients have different functions that we will discuss in the next chapter. Each food can have a different effect on your body depending on its overall nutrient content. The more variety in your diet, the less effect a single food will have on your progress and your health.

Understanding how foods affect us also requires understanding that portion control does not always mean using tiny plates and eating small serving sizes. While a caloric deficit will inevitably result in at least intermittent hunger, you don't have to be starving all the time to lose weight. The secret is filling your diet with high-volume, nutrient-dense foods. High-volume foods stretch your stomach and send signals to your brain indicating that you are full. When your goal is to maintain or gain weight, there is more room to include foods that are low in volume and nutrients, like the occasional cookie or donut.

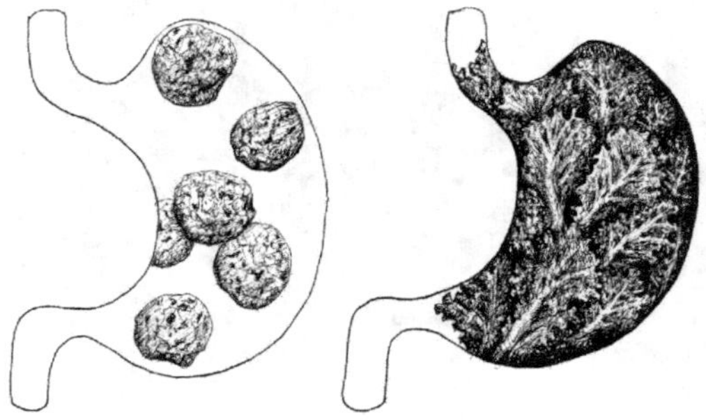

It takes approximately six to eight hours for food to go through our stomach and small intestine before it enters the large intestine. Elimination of undigested waste starts after approximately twenty-four hours. Bodyweight regulation is a very individual process, and it can take different amounts of time to gain or lose fat for different people. What is common among all of us is that a specific food or meal cannot make us healthy or unhealthy, nor can it make us lose weight or gain weight. For example, if we overeat at one meal but not at the next, what would have been stored as fat from the first meal ends up being needed as energy later.

Flexible dieting also involves an understanding that no foods are "good" or "bad," just as no food is "healthy" or "unhealthy." It is what we choose to do with them, i.e. how much and how often we consume them, that can be good or bad. Foods can be nutrient dense or not. "Healthy" means "of good health." Eating birthday cake for every meal can contribute to you becoming unhealthy, but the cake itself is not unhealthy.

Let's consider two different people. The first person claims to eat only whole, unprocessed foods (but she sneaks chocolates from the bowl at work), cooks most of her meals herself, does not track her dietary intake, and works out regularly. The second person eats both whole and processed foods (she even eats a chocolate chip cookie most days), tracks her dietary intake, does not prepare many of her own meals, and works out regularly. The first restricts herself from foods she enjoys, so she ends up mindlessly giving in to temptation to eat foods she thinks are "bad." The second does not feel any guilt over her daily cookie. It makes her happy and is a small enough serving to not have any noticeable effect on her body since her overall calorie and nutrient intake is ideal for her goals. While both approaches have the potential to be successful, the second is much easier for the individual to follow.

Clearly, these are not the only two possible approaches to dieting. There are infinite ways to find your own balance. A flexible dieting approach nourishes both physical and mental health by allowing you to eat the foods that make you feel and perform best. You deserve to be happy, even if you are dieting.

## The Best of Both Worlds

With IIFYM, you can eat whatever you want if it fits within your macronutrient goals for the day. This is great because even though weight is a function of caloric intake, for outcomes like improved body composition and long-term health, macronutrient composition of the diet is critical.

It is a common misconception that IIFYM began in the bodybuilding industry when bodybuilders became tired of eating the same few foods over and over. In truth, the concept of following a macronutrient-based diet is over 120 years old. We have been viewing our food as calories, protein, carbohydrates, and fat since Wilbur Atwater and his colleagues came up with the Atwater system in the late nineteenth century. "IIFYMers" who only pay attention to the macronutrient content of their foods are therefore following a diet that is based on old news. Although the Atwater system is still used to determine the calorie and macronutrient content of foods today, there have been numerous discoveries since Atwater's initial findings that should not be neglected when following a macronutrient-based approach.

In the several decades following the creation of the Atwater system, individuals began to identify and eventually understand another class of nutrients that were present in foods in much smaller quantities than macronutrients: vitamins. (Many minerals had already been discovered, and the public was aware that salt was a necessary nutrient). For example, the discovery of vitamin A was a product of about 130 years of research; in the early 1900s, Elmer McCollum and Marguerite Davis finally "discovered" vitamin A. McCollum and Davis found that rats fed lard and olive oil died while those fed egg or butter extract survived. It turns out that the rats fed lard and olive oil were deficient in vitamin A, which is found in eggs and butter. Based on these findings, McCollum began identifying certain "protective foods" that were supposed to protect against disease because of their vitamin content. To this day, there are still people who adhere to a "protective diet" in hopes of preventing disease.

We now have enough knowledge to understand that food is more than the sum of its nutrient parts. We know that foods can be categorized by macronutrients, water, vitamins, minerals, and phytochemicals. We know that any benefits from food come from consuming an overall balanced diet that has a variety of foods (and therefore a variety of nutrients and other beneficial compounds). To maximize the beneficial impact of our diets on our health, we must consider not only the nutrients in food but also the other aspects of the foods themselves and their relation to our own personal needs and preferences.

While the IIFYM approach sometimes lacks focus on micronutrients and beneficial nonnutritive compounds found in whole foods, a clean eating approach sometimes lacks focus on macronutrients and overall caloric intake. Adhering to one of these approaches without the other can be problematic. Flexible dieting is not an excuse to fill your diet with refined, processed foods and/or foods that are low in nutrients, just as clean eating is not an excuse to go out for a cheat meal on the weekend, be grumpy all the time because you do not allow yourself cheat meals, and not reach your goals because you neglected to pay attention to macronutrient composition.

Clean eating, like any diet that eliminates certain foods, is a luxury. Not all of us have complete control over which foods are accessible. It is much easier to have the freedom of knowing that we can simply consume whichever foods we have access to. Unless you have health reasons that preclude you from being able to eat certain foods, there is no reason to make dieting harder on yourself than it needs to be.

For people who diet to achieve extremely low levels of body fat for bodybuilding or other competitions, eating cold fish, green beans, and sweet potato out of plastic containers is a familiar experience. While this is a great method for sticking to your diet, it is also a great way to become isolated and stressed and to miss out on social and personal pleasures that humans typically associate with eating. There is no logical reason for someone to consume old, cold food in place of a different meal with the same macronutrient composition that is fresh and tastes and smells pleasing.

On the other hand, someone adhering to an IIFYM approach might reach his or her macronutrient goals just fine but meet little to none of his or her micronutrient goals for the day because the person didn't consume enough nutrient-dense choices like fruit and vegetables. A lack of satiating, nutrient-dense foods makes it difficult to stay on track. It is hard to stick to a diet if you never feel satisfied. But even if you do succeed, you might have a difficult time reaching body composition goals (because your body can't pay attention to the processes it should be paying attention to) and maintaining long-term health due to fatigue and inadequate micronutrient intake. Similar problems can arise if we rely on supplements for nutrient "insurance." According to flexible dieting, the base units of our diet are foods and nutrients—not one or the other. Many people act like IIFYM and clean eating contradict each other when in fact they can be viewed as complementary. A simple pairing of these two approaches creates the ideal foundation for success with flexible dieting.

It is a part of normal life to eat for emotional and social reasons, but with today's portion sizes served in American restaurants and prepackaged meals, quantity of food can get out of hand if we don't have self-imposed guidelines. Flexible dieting allows for emotional and social eating if it fits within our numerical guidelines. Because hormones impact on desires and behaviors, we don't want to go out of control with foods that trigger behaviors that will take us outside of our guidelines. A taste of something sweet can either satisfy a craving or create an even stronger craving. It is critical to find your own balance and to allow yourself flexibility without straying too far from your guidelines.

To be successful incorporating these two approaches together, remember that the goal is to take care of ourselves. We want to get most of our calories from nutrient-dense food, but we also want to be able to participate in fulfilling social and cultural activities.

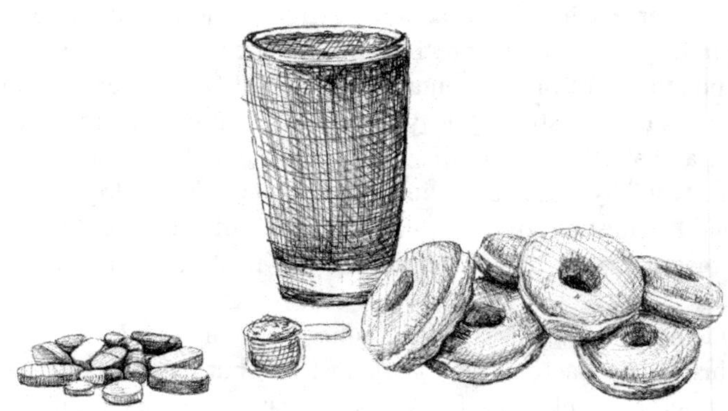

# Don't Trust the Human Brain

Few of us have the willpower to make logical decisions about what to eat. Those of us who do may argue that food is fuel for our bodies and should be treated singularly as such. But regardless of how much willpower one has, palatability will always compete with the "food is fuel" concept.

Many packaged foods are engineered to maximize palatability. Palatability is a pleasure derived from a food or beverage that satisfies our taste. Palatability encourages us to eat enough to meet our bodies' needs, but in modern-day America, where there are so many inexpensive, highly palatable foods, we are often encouraged to eat much more than what our body needs. If something tastes good and is enjoyable to you, and if your brain is telling you that it is rewarding and pleasurable, why wouldn't you want more?

In the absence of numerical dietary guidelines, we are left to trust ourselves to eat the right foods in the right amounts. Unfortunately, many of us cannot compete with the excessive availability of palatable foods. Others of us hate to reward ourselves with palatable foods, so we severely restrict or even prohibit ourselves from enjoying them.

At certain restaurants and social gatherings, it can be difficult to find foods that are dense in nutrients rather than palatability. Palatability of a specific food decreases when satiety sets in, so when we eat foods that aren't very satiating—for example, foods that are low in fiber and protein—the perceived need for palatability typically remains high.

Although many of us lack the willpower and/or knowledge necessary to eat the right foods in the proper amounts to reach our goals, many of us have the willpower and/or knowledge necessary to stick to a budget. With numerical guidelines written out for us, half the battle of making logical decisions about food is already won. Once we have spelled out how much we need to eat and which types of foods will get us there, we are left with one last decision: which of these foods do we choose? It turns out that you can do very well no matter what decisions you make if the total nutrient content of your diet fits in these guidelines.

With flexible dieting, when and what we eat is guided by a set of numbers. Some foods taste good; they make us want to eat more and more of them. Other foods are less palatable, but we know that we can get necessary nutrients from them. Flexible dieting sets up parameters for protein, carbohydrates, fat, and micronutrients (vitamins and minerals). We can make decisions within these parameters however we want. We don't have to worry about eating when we're hungry and stopping when we're full. We don't have to worry about what foods are "good" or "bad" for our goals. We just need to stick to our budget.

The human brain is programmed to overeat. When we already have sufficient energy, there is no regulation system in place to tell us not to grab another french fry or bite of dessert. An effective way to "reprogram" our decision making about what to eat is to impose a set of rules that we must follow. We follow rules at work and in school, so why don't we respect rules when it comes to our health? The rule of flexible dieting is simple: fulfill macronutrient requirements by eating anything you want as long as your overall diet is high in nutrient-dense foods.

While keeping a diet high in variety helps to ensure that we get adequate nutrients, research suggests that the more the variety of foods available, the more that we eat. This is often referred to as the "buffet effect." But as an external regulation system, flexible dieting allows us to take some of whatever we want from the buffet as long as the portions add up correctly and fit our guidelines.

Many proponents of flexible dieting love to cite research and explain why a flexible dieting approach is better than other dietary approaches, but when we focus on the scientific evidence, we often forget that the psychological component is just as important. Taking care of your mental health by adhering to a holistic approach is critical for long-term success on a diet. If you follow your diet perfectly yet you are miserable, there is a better approach out there. You are a human, not a science experiment. It is for this reason that I have decided to refrain from citing specific research studies in this book. Science is the foundation, but you are the art.

# 3
# MACRONUTRIENTS

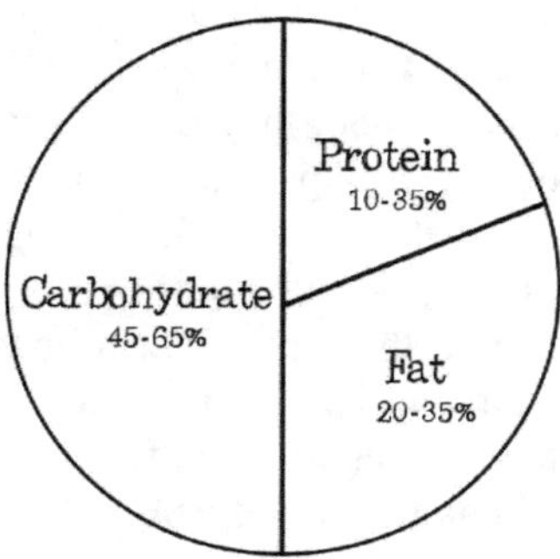


Macronutrients ("macros"), or nutrients that we require in large quantities, include fat, protein, and carbohydrates. Alcohol is also technically a macronutrient, but we will not discuss it in this chapter. Macronutrients make up approximately 90% of the dry weight of our food. All three macronutrients supply us with energy needed for normal functions. Fats can be saturated, monounsaturated, or polyunsaturated. Trans fats also exist but are not beneficial for human consumption. Carbohydrates include various types of sugars, and protein is made up of amino acids. The USDA recommends that adults consume a diet with the following macronutrient composition: 45–65% carbohydrates, 10–35% protein, and 20–35% fat. Because each of these macronutrients plays unique, critical roles in our bodies, adjusting the macronutrient composition of our diet will have a direct effect on our body composition, athletic performance, and overall health.

## Carbohydrates

Carbohydrates are our bodies' main sources of fuel. Physical activity, brain function, gut health, waste elimination, and normal operation of our organs all depend on the presence of adequate carbohydrates in our bodies.

The carbohydrates on nutrition labels are broken down into fiber, sugar, and sugar alcohols. What is not explicitly mentioned is the "other" carbohydrate category, which represents starch. Starch, which is typically the most common carbohydrate in human diets, consists of glucose molecules joined by glycosidic bonds. Root vegetables, legumes, and grains are excellent sources of starch. Their digestibility is increased when cooked, and therefore, raw starch sources are much more difficult to digest than cooked starch sources. Think of a raw potato vs. a cooked potato. Resistant starch, found mostly in raw starch sources, is largely indigestible by humans and functions like a soluble, fermentable fiber.

The difference between whole grains and refined grains is that only whole grains provide the bran, germ, and endosperm, while refined grains lack the bran and germ and therefore contain less fiber, vitamins, and essential fatty acids. However, many refined grain products are enriched to replace nutrients lost during processing.

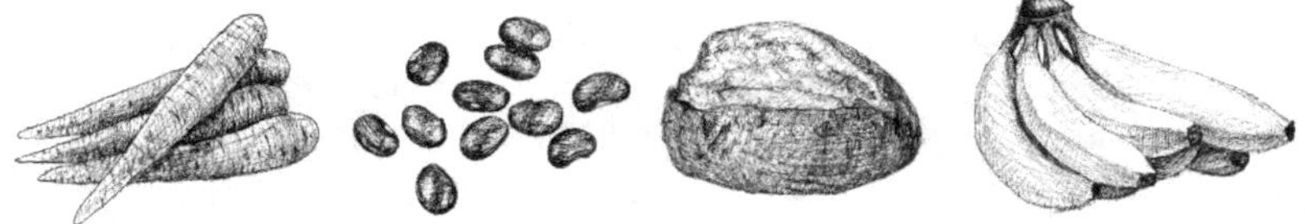

Sugar is typically grouped into naturally occurring sugars, such as those found naturally in fruit and milk, and sugars that are added during processing. Sugars can be further categorized into monosaccharides (glucose, fructose, galactose), disaccharides (lactose, maltose, sucrose, etc.), and oligosaccharides. Molecules with greater than nine carbons, or polysaccharides, are starches. Smaller sugar molecules are generally digested more rapidly than starches, although factors like fiber, protein, and fat content of the rest of a meal can affect absorption rate. Once consumed, starch and sugar are both broken down into glucose, raising blood sugar levels. More about the effect of carbohydrates on blood sugar levels is discussed later in the "Meal Timing" chapter.

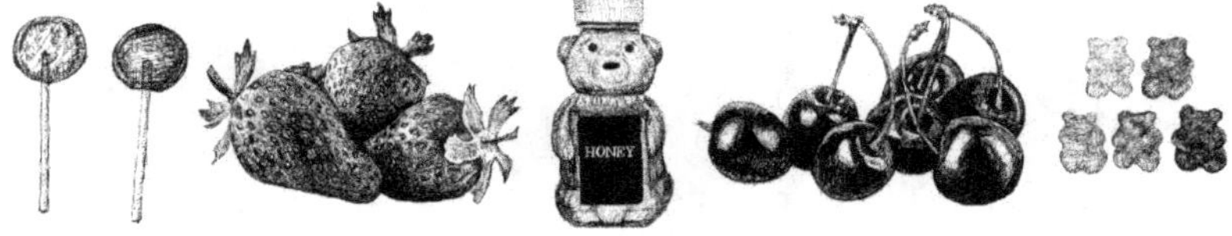

Fiber, which occurs naturally only in plant sources, is a largely indigestible carbohydrate that is associated with digestive health and several positive health outcomes. Soluble fiber, like gums, pectins, beta-glucans, and psyllium, dissolves in water in the gastrointestinal (GI)

tract to form a gel-like substance and can reduce blood sugar levels. Insoluble fiber, like lignin and cellulose, does not dissolve in water and passes through the GI tract in bulk form. Insoluble fiber can increase the rate at which food and waste travel through your GI tract. Some fibers are fermentable in the GI tract, meaning that gut bacteria can ferment them and use them for fuel. Beans and legumes are common sources of fermentable fibers. The USDA recommends that adults consume at least 25–30 grams of fiber per day.

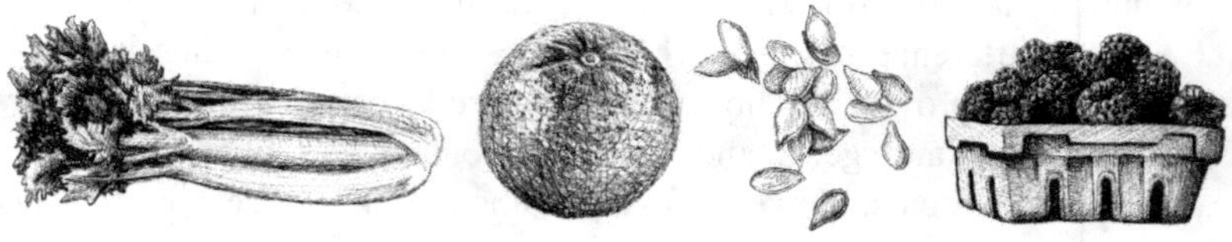

Nutritionally speaking, carbohydrates are broken down into starch, sugar, and fiber. However, sugar alcohols are consumed by many individuals and included in many processed foods to reduce their added sugar content. Sugar alcohols are often listed on nutrition labels with carbohydrates and contain zero to three calories per gram, whereas carbohydrates contain an average of four calories per gram. Sugar alcohols include erythritol, isomalt, hydrogenated starch hydrolysates, lactitol, mannitol, maltitol, sorbitol, and xylitol. They do not increase blood glucose levels as much as other carbohydrates do.

Sugar substitutes are not carbohydrates but are often used to decrease the carbohydrate and caloric content of a food while giving it a sweeter taste. The FDA has approved the following sugar substitutes for human consumption: acesulfame potassium (i.e. acesulfame K), advantame, aspartame, neotame, saccharin, and sucralose. These are typically mentioned in ingredient lists but not listed on nutrition labels themselves because they contain negligible calories in portions that are typically consumed.


# Fat

"Lipid" is the correct term for what we refer to as dietary "fat." Technically, oils are liquid at room temperature, while fats are usually solid at room temperature, but when we talk about the macronutrients, we use the term "fat" to denote all lipids. (In the US, nutrition labels list "fat" rather than "lipid" content.) Dietary fats, or triglycerides, are composed of fatty acids and glycerol.

In the body, fatty acids, triglycerides, and cholesterol provide energy storage, protect our organs, aid in the absorption of fat-soluble vitamins, and act as messengers for proteins. Fat also functions as a backup source of fuel when carbohydrates are not available. Very low-fat diets can suppress hormone levels and impair absorption of fat-soluble vitamins A, D, E, and K.

Fatty acids are typically classified by both structure and length. Structurally, fatty acids can be unsaturated or saturated. The carbon chains of unsaturated fat molecules are not completely saturated with hydrogen atoms. In other words, not all carbons are bonded to the maximum possible number of hydrogen atoms.

Monounsaturated fatty acids (MUFAs) have only one double bond, giving them a lower melting point than saturated fats but a higher melting point than polyunsaturated fatty acids (PUFAs), which have two or more double bonds. MUFAs are found in olive oil, peanut oil, canola oil, avocados, most nuts, and high-oleic safflower and sunflower oils.

PUFAs, alpha-linolenic acid (an omega-3 fatty acid) and linoleic acid (an omega-6 fatty acid), are considered essential fatty acids (EFAs) because the human body cannot synthesize them on its own. PUFAs help build cell membranes and nerve coverings, reduce inflammation, move muscles, clot blood, and may be protective against heart disease. Sources of omega-3 PUFAs include fatty fish, walnuts, flaxseeds, chia seeds, canola oil, and unhydrogenated soybean oil. Sources of omega-6 PUFAs include corn, safflower, soybean, sunflower, and walnut oils.

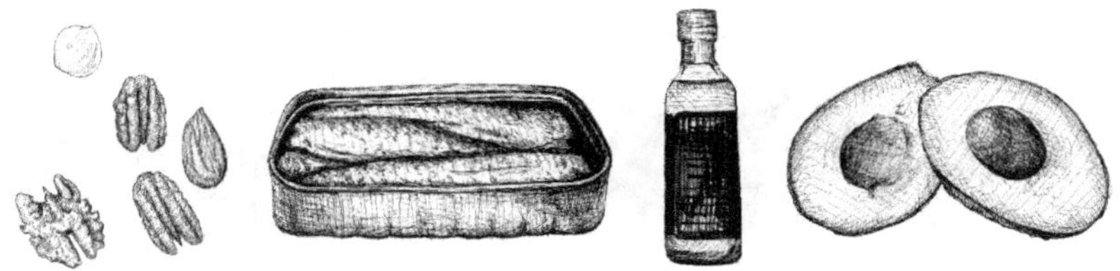

Saturated fat molecules are saturated with hydrogen atoms, meaning that they hold as many hydrogen atoms as they possibly can. Saturated fatty acids are solid at room temperature and are commonly found in red meat, full-fat dairy products, cheese, and coconut oil. Data on high saturated fat intake provide mixed outcomes. Claims now exist that saturated fat intake does not necessarily lead to an increased risk of heart disease as was once thought; however, research suggests that a high ratio of saturated fat intake to unsaturated fat intake could have negative health effects. The 2015–2020 Dietary Guidelines recommend limiting saturated fat intake to 10% of one's total calorie intake. For 2,000 daily calories, this is 22.2 g a day, which is nearly fourteen eggs' worth!

A high ratio of unsaturated fat to saturated fat intake has been shown to lower LDL cholesterol and triglyceride levels. Saturated fat itself is not inherently bad, but a high ratio of saturated fat to unsaturated fat intake may be associated with risk factors of heart disease, such as increased LDL cholesterol levels.

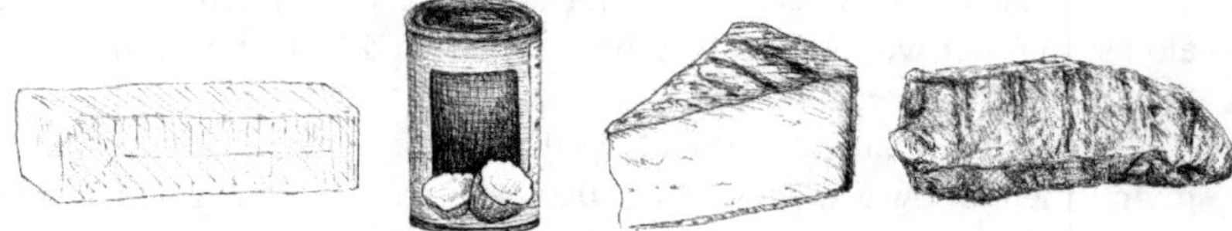

Natural trans fat comes only from ruminant animals (e.g. cattle, sheep, and goats) and is formed when bacteria in their stomachs digest grass. There is a lack of evidence that these are harmful. Man-made trans fats are a byproduct of hydrogenation, which is the process of turning oils into solid fats. There are no known benefits to consuming artificial trans fat. Trans fats have been banned by the U.S. Food and Drug Administration (FDA). Even a small amount of trans-fatty acid in the diet may be associated with inflammation and insulin resistance, which can lead to chronic conditions like heart disease and diabetes.

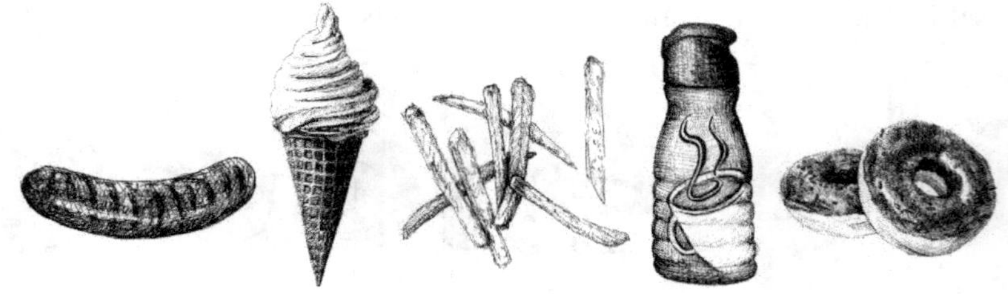

When categorized by length, fatty acids can be short-chain fatty acids (SCFAs; less than six carbons), medium-chain fatty acids (MCFAs; six to twelve carbons), long-chain fatty acids (LCFAs; thirteen to twenty-one carbons), or very-long-chain fatty acids (VLCFAs; twenty-two carbons or longer). SCFAs and MCFAs are largely absorbed through the portal vein; longer chains must first be packed into chylomicrons, which are lipoproteins consisting mostly of triglycerides that enter lymphatic capillaries and are absorbed into the blood through the subclavian vein.

SCFAs are mainly produced by fermentation of soluble fiber in the large intestine but can be consumed directly through food sources as well.

## Protein

Protein consists of one or more chains of amino acid residues and plays important roles in tissue repair, enzyme and hormone production, DNA replication, and transporting molecules. Protein is found in hair, skin, nails, bone, and muscle. Dietary protein helps to preserve and build muscle.

High-protein diets are effective at reducing body fat, specifically abdominal fat. Protein is the most satiating macronutrient, and protein has the highest thermic effect of food (TEF), which is the energy required to digest and absorb food. The thermic effect of protein (20–30%) is much higher than that of carbohydrates (5–10%) or fat (0–3%). High protein intake can also increase levels of appetite-reducing hormones (GLP-1, leptin, PYY, CCK) and decrease levels of the hunger hormone, ghrelin.

Amino acids are the building blocks of protein. A compound made up of two or more amino acids is called a peptide. A chain of ten or more peptides is a protein; proteins made up of ten to fifty peptides are also called polypeptides. Because proteins are made up of amino acids, they are often classified by which amino acids are contained within them. Complete proteins contain all the amino acids required for your body to build new proteins, while incomplete proteins lack one or more of these essential amino acids. Animal and soy products tend to have complete proteins, while most plant products have incomplete proteins.

Can you get all amino acids from plants? Some plant sources like chia and hemp seeds are complete proteins, but keep in mind that amino acids can form complete proteins in the body even if a single food does not contain all the essential amino acids. As we have seen time and time again, nutrition is a matter of balance. Eating a variety of foods will help to ensure you are getting adequate nutrients. For vegetarians and vegans, consuming grains and legumes regularly can ensure adequate intake of all amino acids. However, there is no reason to eat grains and legumes at the same time to form a complete protein. Your body will manage just fine if you eat them at different times.

There are four levels of protein structure. The linear sequence of amino acid residues forms the primary structure. The secondary structure can be formed into alpha helices or beta sheets, and the tertiary structure describes how these helices or sheets are folded into a globular structure.

The subunits (single protein molecules) fit together in a quaternary structure.

When we heat or cook proteins, the structure unfolds in a process called denaturation. Nutritional value remains unchanged, however. The primary structure is not affected by denaturation, meaning that the amino acids are not destroyed. Our stomach acid will denature proteins even if our cooking method does not.

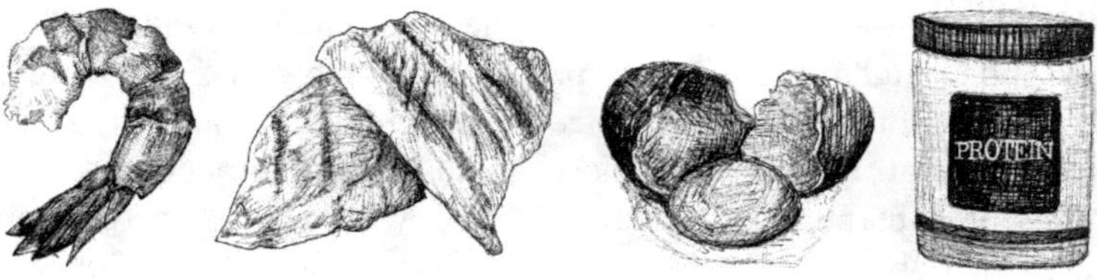


## Putting It All Together

Just as no food is inherently bad, none of the macronutrients are inherently bad. Unfortunately, we often fear eating too much of one macronutrient because it seems like an easy fix to simply restrict one of the three macronutrients. Consequently, the most popular diets are often low-carbohydrate and low-fat diets. Many people even fear consumption of "too much protein." While it is certainly possible to consume more nutrients than what is required to meet your goals, too much of any one macronutrient is not necessarily a negative on its own. In some cases, you can follow a diet that restricts or eliminates one macronutrient and still overdo it on one or both the other two. However, you will also probably encounter side effects from not getting enough of the macronutrient that you are avoiding.

To determine exactly how your macronutrient consumption will affect your physique and health, you need to look at the bigger picture: your overall caloric intake. A caloric surplus will surely make you gain weight, so if your goal is to lose weight, and you are consuming more calories than you require to maintain your weight, then you will not achieve your goal. However, if you are consuming 80% of your calories from carbohydrates in the form of anything from vegetables to cereal to gummy bears, then you can still lose fat if your overall caloric intake is less than what is required for you to maintain your weight. This is why restrictive diets like the jelly bean diet can result in weight loss.

There are many factors to consider when determining an appropriate macronutrient ratio for your diet, including current diet composition, physical activity routine, health diagnoses, and food intolerances or allergies. What might be an appropriate macronutrient composition for one person might not work for another. Be careful following generic calorie or macronutrient requirements because we each have unique health situations and goals, and we don't all respond to diet changes the same way. Sometimes it takes weeks or months of flexible dieting to be able to predict how you will respond to dietary adjustments.

People with specific medical diagnoses may require unique macronutrient ratios. While protein does not harm kidneys or liver or bones in healthy individuals with balanced diets, extremely high-protein diets are not recommended for individuals who have kidney problems or who have been fasting for a long time. Carbohydrates should make up a large portion of the diet for most individuals, but individuals with conditions like insulin resistance, diabetes, or metabolic syndrome might need to be particularly careful about carbohydrate consumption and the glycemic index of the carbohydrates that they choose to consume. Fat is an essential part of the diet for all of us, but individuals with certain digestive conditions like Crohn's disease might need to limit their fat intake. These are just a few examples of how an appropriate macronutrient composition of one's diet can vary from person to person. Individuals should consult with their physicians prior to initiating any diet program.

## Water

Water is required for us to absorb each of the three macronutrients. Water lacks nutritional value itself, although minerals like calcium, sodium, and magnesium can be found in water. The daily Adequate Intake (AI) of water is 3 liters for men and 2.2 liters for women. If you are active, you may want to increase water and electrolyte intake to replace what is lost in sweat and breath. It is not uncommon for very active individuals to drink 6 to 8 liters of water or more per day. Dehydration can lead to countless issues, from decreased athletic performance, mood deviations, and memory loss to increased anxiety and fatigue.

Tracking water intake is not a fundamental component of flexible dieting, but if you struggle to drink enough, you can track consumption until you get into a routine of drinking more. If you have no idea how much water you drink, it might also be a good idea to track your intake for at least a few days to get a more complete picture. The more you know about your intake and exercise, the better you can tailor your diet to your current situation to maximize results in the future.

## Micronutrients

Micronutrients are substances that we require in much smaller amounts than macronutrients. Micronutrients include all the vitamins and minerals that we need to live. Many flexible dieters track macronutrients to the exact gram or to a range of grams but don't track micronutrients the same way. With flexible dieting, the goal is to consume adequate amounts of micronutrients while following your guidelines for macronutrients and enjoying your life. If your diet is at a caloric deficit, then it can be difficult to get adequate nutrients since you are not giving your body enough to maintain its current weight. If your diet is at a caloric surplus, you will have an easier time reaching adequate micronutrient intake, assuming your diet is balanced and varied. Nutrient-dense foods will give you the most "bang for your buck," that is, they will have a higher nutrient-to-calorie ratio. When you hear the term "empty calories," it is referring to the opposite situation, or foods that are low in nutrients for how many calories they contain.

As with water, it might be a good idea to track your micronutrient intake until you develop a sense of what your current micronutrient intake looks like. Once you know whether you struggle to get enough of certain micronutrients, you can decide whether regularly tracking micronutrient intake is helpful for you.

# 4

## CALCULATING YOUR MACRONUTRIENT-INTAKE GOALS

You may or may not have seen someone share his or her calculated macronutrients or "macros." An example set of macros might be written as 50f/250c/150p. What does this mean? It means that this person is aiming to consume 50 g of fat, 250 g of carbohydrates, and 150 g of protein each day. The numbers in this example are arbitrary. Let's discuss how you can determine your own daily macronutrient intake.

Before we get into all the guesswork required in calculating your numbers, let's discuss one of the most important prerequisites, which is a component that many people omit from their calculations. This prerequisite is to track your dietary intake before you ever start sticking to any set numbers. Write down everything you eat for at least three days. Keep track of calories and grams of fat, carbohydrates, and protein since these are what you will be calculating. Once you have an idea of how much food you are eating, you are ready to compare those numbers to numbers that you will obtain from inputting some of your information into formulas. Since this chapter is about calculating your macronutrient intake goals, we will first review the process for making calculations.

There are two parts to calculating your macronutrient goals: (1) making initial calculations and (2) tweaking those calculations based on experience. You can use an online calculator to find your macronutrient intake goals, but if you ignore the second step, you are missing out on the advantage of human intelligence and the fact that each individual's metabolism is unique. If you estimate your macronutrient intake goals based on experience without performing a calculation, you are missing out on the advantage that mathematics offers. You might notice that the calculations involve a lot of guesswork and manipulation because everyone is different. Because of this, "cookie-cutter" diet plans cannot give the best results. Keep in mind that you should check with your doctor or health professional before starting any diet, flexible dieting or otherwise. If you have a specific diet recommended by a doctor or professional, you should adhere to that advice and incorporate flexible dieting into your approach with proper supervision.

At best, calculating your macronutrient intake goals gives you a rough idea of what someone with your measurements and lifestyle should be eating to reach your fitness goals. Calculations based on formulas can never accurately represent what you personally should be eating to reach your goals; however, a calculated estimate is much better than a shot in the dark. Once you have estimated calories and broken them down into macronutrients, you can tweak them based on knowledge and experience. Then, the process of personalizing your macronutrient intake goals continues beyond the first set of calculations. After you try sticking to your new diet for a couple of weeks, you can tweak your macronutrient intake goals based on how your weight is changing (or not changing), how well you are able to adhere to the diet, how you are feeling, and any other changes in variables that might arise.

## Calories

Let's start by estimating a daily caloric intake that can get you on track to reaching your goals. If you can take measurements using laboratory equipment, you may be able to calculate your metabolic rate and energy expenditure. Basal metabolic rate (BMR) can be measured through gas analysis via indirect or direct calorimetry and requires a resting but awake state in which the sympathetic nervous system is not stimulated. Resting metabolic rate (RMR) can be measured under less strict conditions. Energy expenditure can be measured with an open-circuit indirect calorimeter that requires a mask, hood, canopy, or even a closed chamber, where subjects are confined during their stay. In more normal living environments, doubly labeled water (DLW), or water in which hydrogens and oxygens are replaced with isotopes, must be used so that expenditure can be traced.

If you don't have access to calorimeters or doubly labeled water, then let's make some calculations. Many online calculators (like the one available at acadiafit.com) use an approach that is similar to the one we will walk through. If you want to make the calculations yourself, or if you are interested in finding out how to make the calculations, then keep reading. If not, feel free to skip ahead.

The process of estimating your BMR and total daily energy expenditure (TDEE) involves both math and guesswork. TDEE is made up of resting energy expenditure (REE), which refers to the BMR, and non-resting energy expenditure (NREE), which includes exercise activity thermogenesis (EAT), nonexercise activity thermogenesis (NEAT), and the thermic effect of food (TEF).

The first step to figuring out your TDEE is to estimate your basal metabolic rate (BMR). The Mifflin St. Jeor formula is generally recognized as the most accurate formula for this, but there are other formulas that provide similar results.

<u>For males:</u>

$$9.99 \times \text{weight (kg)} + 6.25 \times \text{height (cm)} - 4.92 \times \text{age (years)} + 5 = \text{BMR}$$

<u>For females:</u>

$$9.99 \times \text{weight (kg)} + 6.25 \times \text{height (cm)} - 4.92 \times \text{age (years)} - 161 = \text{BMR}$$

The Harris-Benedict formula was revised by Mifflin and St. Jeor in 1990 to come up with the above equation. Before that, the most recent version was revised by Roza and Shizgal in 1984:

<u>For males:</u>

$$88.362 + 13.397 \times \text{weight (kg)} + 4.799 \times \text{height (cm)} - 5.677 \times \text{age (years)} = \text{BMR}$$

<u>For females:</u>

$$447.593 + 9.247 \times \text{weight (kg)} + 3.098 \times \text{height (cm)} - 4.330 \times \text{age (years)} = \text{BMR}$$

Although the Mifflin St. Jeor formula is commonly used, you might notice that lean body mass is missing from the formula. Research has shown that we can accurately predict metabolic rate without any information about body composition. Most of our TDEE comes from heart, lungs, kidneys, brain, and liver. Organs burn more calories at rest than muscle, but muscle comparatively burns more calories during activity. If you know your lean mass weight or percentage body fat, feel free to use a different equation. If you have no idea, we can tweak our estimation once we get to the experience component of the estimation process.

The Katch-McArdle formula accounts for lean body mass and is designed to estimate BMR, while the Cunningham formula accounts for lean body mass but is designed to estimate RMR. Note that lean body mass = body weight – body fat.

<u>Katch McArdle:</u> $\text{BMR} = 370 + 21.6 \times \text{lean body mass (kg)}$

<u>Cunningham:</u> $\text{RMR} = 500 + 22 \times \text{lean body mass (kg)}$

The metabolic rate calculated from the above equations represents how many calories you would burn if you were figuratively a potato. Thus, these calculations determine how many calories you would need to consume to maintain your weight (if you were figuratively a potato). So let's multiply by a factor to estimate NREE. You may have used a fitness tracker that tells you how many calories you burned in a day. While these trackers are not entirely accurate, they do provide an estimation from which to make comparisons. We burn calories when we exercise, when we do any activity at all, and when our body completes its normal involuntary functions, such as breathing. If you don't know how many calories you burn per day, then you need to multiply by an estimation factor. Even if you do know how many calories you burn, the number of calories you burn today will not be the same number of calories you burn tomorrow or next Friday. I doubt you will want to make a separate calculation for every day of your life, so let's estimate.

Consider how you spend most of your time. Are you usually sitting or standing? Do you run around all day carrying heavy equipment as part of your job? Now consider your exercise regimen. Can you hold a conversation while exercising, or can you barely catch your breath?

Now do your best to find an "average." For example, if you work at a desk job or sit on the couch most of the time but do extremely intense workouts for forty-five minutes on five days per week, even though you may be improving your body composition and look great, your overall lifestyle can probably be characterized as lightly active.

Understand that this calculation requires making an educated guess about an average of all your time, both awake and asleep. The alternative is to use a fitness tracker. You may need to adjust these numbers once you get started and see how your body responds. Even if you sit on the couch all day every day, multiply by 1.2.

<u>Not active</u>: Multiply by 1.2

<u>Lightly active</u>: Multiply by 1.375

<u>Moderately active</u>: Multiply by 1.55

<u>Very active</u>: Multiply by 1.725

<u>Extremely active</u>: Multiply by 1.9

Part of the complication of calculating your own macronutrient intake is that you need to be honest with yourself; however, one of the benefits is that you can customize your approach. For example, if you want an aggressive approach for losing weight, underestimate your expenditure.

The final step for calculating your ideal caloric intake is to adjust the number you have calculated according to your goals. Now that we have determined where you are now, think about where you want to be. Multiply by a factor depending on how aggressive of an approach you want to take.

**Lose Fat** : Multiply by 0.75 - 0.85

**Maintain** : Multiply 1

**Gain Muscle** : Multiply by 1.05 - 1.15

These numbers are not special. The idea is to simply choose a pace that at first isn't too aggressive.

The final step to estimate your recommended caloric intake is to factor in your current dietary intake. Try tracking everything you eat for a few days or a week without changing anything. If you already know that your current intake is extremely lower or higher than the number you have calculated, start with something in the middle of the two. For instance, if your goal is to lose fat and you calculated 2,500 calories when your current caloric intake is 2,000 calories, you might want to readjust. Just because you calculated that someone with your gender, age, height, and weight should consume this number doesn't mean that the calculation produces a result that is best for you. Your BMR might be extremely high or low for someone with your demographic information. We will further discuss the idea of tweaking based on experience later.

## Macronutrients

Now that you have calculated a set number of calories, it is time to break that number down into macronutrients. As previously mentioned, the Institute of Medicine (IOM) recommends that 45–65% of energy come from carbohydrates, 10–35% of energy come from protein, and 20–35% of energy come from fat. These Acceptable Macronutrient Distribution Ranges (AMDRs) are percentages of total energy intake suggested for each macronutrient. Many people favor a lower-carb approach for fat loss and a higher-carb approach for muscle gain, but your personal macronutrient split depends on your metabolism, exercise regimen, and preference. While a high-protein diet is beneficial for many people, those in a severe caloric deficit and with very low levels of body fat will require higher-protein intake to keep carbohydrate and fat intake lower, which should help maximize satiety and fat loss.

Optimizing protein intake is critical for success because of its satiating potential and its ability to preserve or build lean body mass. But how much do you need? Research indicates that 1.8 g/kg body weight (0.82 g/lb body weight—because in the US we do silly things like combining metric and imperial measures) is enough for strength athletes and any active individuals who are restricting calories.

Although a protein intake higher than 0.82 g/lb of body weight might not have any effect on body composition, a higher protein intake can be beneficial if it promotes diet adherence or encourages an overall balanced diet. Protein will help you feel fuller for a longer period of time than the same number of calories in carbohydrates and/or fat; this is perhaps the best reason to increase protein above 0.82 g/lb. Calories must come from somewhere, so if you are trying to gain muscle and have all these carbohydrates and fat in your budget to "spend," it might be more tempting to opt for low-nutrient foods simply because you have more available to you. Higher-protein intake reduces appetite and has a beneficial impact on weight-regulating hormones. Because of its high TEF, a high-protein diet that has the same number of calories as a lower-protein diet can also slightly increase metabolic rate.

Appropriate fat and carbohydrate intakes are affected by factors like insulin sensitivity, gender, activity level, type of activity performed, and personal preference. More active individuals will require more carbohydrates than less active individuals. Endurance athletes will require more carbohydrates than strength athletes. Higher estrogen in a female might mean greater reliance on fats than carbohydrates compared to a male with otherwise similar age, height, weight, body type, and goals. Insulin-resistant individuals may have better results on a lower-carbohydrate diet that does not cause large fluctuations in blood-sugar or insulin levels.

Of all the factors that can affect which macronutrient ratio will work best for you, perhaps one of the most important is the potential for adherence. If you have trouble sticking to a low-carbohydrate or low-fat diet, then it does not make sense for you.

If you have no idea where to begin, you can try establishing a target for fat intake in the middle of the IOM recommendations, at 27.5% of your caloric intake. Then the guideline for carbohydrates can be set after protein and fat allocation targets are set. You can compare this with your current intake and see if you tend to favor a higher-carbohydrate or a higher-fat approach. Once you track your current dietary intake for a few days to see where you are, you can meet somewhere in the middle of what one might estimate based on your situation and goals and what you are currently doing. For example, if your diet is too high in calories and full of carbohydrate-rich snacks, and you are not very active, you might want to swap some carbohydrates out for protein and fat while decreasing your overall caloric intake.

We discussed protein calculated in grams, but how do we get from the IOM recommended percentages to gram amounts for each macronutrient? Differences in the heat of combustion of distinct types of the same macronutrient exist but are generally ignored. For instance, monosaccharides have 3.75 kcal/g, while disaccharides have 3.95 kcal/g, and polysaccharides have 4.15–4.20 kcal/g. These differences are so small that they are considered equivalent, which is a source of error in tracking dietary intake. Nevertheless, the following Atwater factors are commonly used to indicate how much energy is provided by each macronutrient:

Protein = 4 calories / gram

Carbohydrate = 4 calories / gram

Fat = 9 calories / gram

Let's try a simple calculation using someone who weighs 150 lb and has calculated a need for 2,000 calories per day. At 1 g protein per lb of body weight, he or she will need 150 g of protein per day.

If we use 25% of the diet being composed of dietary fat, we get (0.25)(2,000 calories) = 500 calories per day from fat. Fat is 9 calories per gram, and 500 calories/9 calories per gram = 55.6 grams of fat per day.

Now let's fill in the rest with carbohydrates; 2,000 calories − 500 calories from fat = 1,500 calories leftover. With 150 g of protein per day, 150 g × 4 calories/gram = 600 calories from protein, which leaves us with 2,000 − 500 − 600 calories = 900 calories per day from carbohydrates, and 900 calories/4 calories per gram = 225 g of carbohydrates per day.

The final step is to set ranges around the numbers you have calculated. Nutrition data are never entirely accurate, so you do not have to worry about tracking your intake to the exact gram unless you enjoy doing so. The individual in our example might aim for a daily intake of 145–155 g protein, 52.6–58.6 g fat, and 220–230 g carbohydrates, for example.

## Micronutrients

There are no formulas to calculate micronutrient intake for individuals given height, weight, age, and gender since we lack enough data on each micronutrient to do this, but the USDA has established recommendations for individuals by age group. However, each individual may require specific, personalized recommendations based on genetic and lifestyle factors.

## The Experience Component

As you can see, finding an appropriate calorie intake and macronutrient composition of your diet to meet your goals requires more guesswork than calculation. And now that we have gone through all the calculating and estimating, it is time to tweak even further based on individual experience. The first step to the experience component is to adjust based on past experiences, and the next step, later, is to tweak as you gain even more experience with yourself. This is a journey. It is likely that your starting calorie and macronutrient guidelines will not be perfect, so do not worry if after the first week you are not seeing the progress that you had been hoping for. Success with flexible dieting comes from getting continuous feedback from your body and adjusting your dietary intake goals appropriately.

What works best in theory does not always work best in practice because life is not a lab. To maximize success with flexible dieting, you need to understand and apply scientific evidence, but you also need to know how to look at yourself as the unique individual that you are. Flexible dieting is about more than calculating and finding the perfect macronutrient ratio; it is also about understanding yourself and your body. This cannot be done at one time point. It takes time to observe feedback and progress, to make changes when necessary, and to see the results add up over a period of time.

It is important to check your weight and body measurements and take pictures of yourself as you progress so that you can effectively measure progress and tweak your intake goals as necessary. Do not act based on your weight the first day after you start your new diet. Daily fluctuations are normal. Weigh yourself once a week, or weigh yourself every day but only use the average weight over the course of each week as data points. As you get to know your own metabolism, it will become easier to anticipate how your body will react to dietary changes.

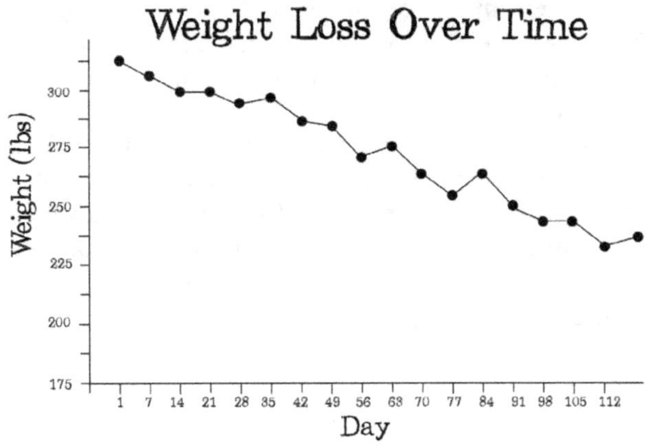


Two people in the same caloric deficit or surplus will likely lose or gain weight at very different rates. See how your body responds over the first few weeks, and go from there once you know what your body is capable of.

## Summary

How to estimate your appropriate calorie and macronutrient intake:
1. Use a commonly accepted equation to calculate your calorie intake recommendations. If you have access to personalized testing, you can get an even more personalized result.
2. Determine an appropriate macronutrient composition of your diet by examining your own personal situation and goals. Use Atwater factors to convert from calories to grams.
3. Check your progress at regular intervals, and adjust your intake as necessary to maximize progress.

Before you start following a specific dietary approach, it is necessary to check with a physician or other health professional to investigate family history and see which diagnoses you have now or are at risk for. Healthy individuals with no major diagnoses may not require special dietary guidelines, but those of us with diagnoses might. It is important to check with your doctor to see if he or she has any specific recommendations for you.

Calculating macronutrient intake is not a one-time event. No matter how accurate you think your calculation is, you will need to adjust as your body changes over time. A key strength of flexible dieting is that your diet can continue to evolve with you, allowing you to not only reach your goals but also to surpass them and accomplish things you might have never thought you could have.

As you will learn throughout this book, it is impossible to precisely track dietary intake. There are factors outside of our control that we cannot account for, from inaccurate nutrition labels to varying water content in a potato. If you track your dietary intake with the goal of getting within a small range of grams for your macronutrients, then you are being as accurate as life will allow.

# 5
# TRACKING YOUR DIETARY INTAKE

The first step to tracking your macronutrient intake is developing a broad understanding of what the macronutrient content of various foods looks like. If you skip this step, you will not be able to brainstorm meal ideas in your head. Instead, you will have to search foods in a database or Google them to figure out what their macronutrient content looks like before you can decide what to eat (or what "fits your macros"). Start by thinking of all your favorite foods. What do you normally eat in a day? What do you want to eat in a day? Now let's see where they fall in the diagram below:

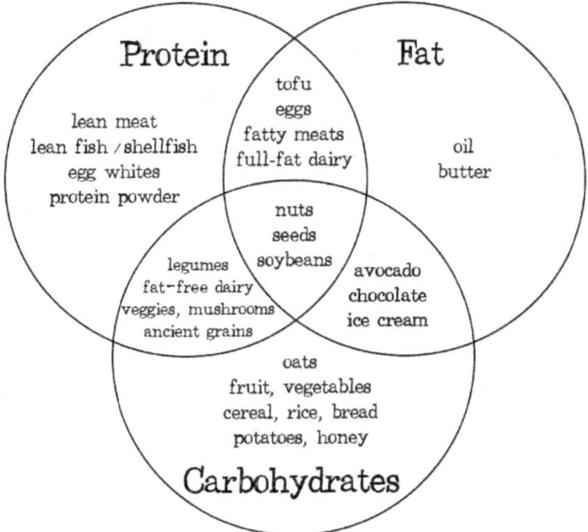


As you get started with tracking your intake, ask yourself the following questions: What fits my plan? What do I need to cut back on? What do I need more of to optimize my progress?

The purpose of having numeric goals with flexible dieting is not to cause stress about hitting these numbers to the exact gram and feel like a failure if we do not. Rather, the idea is that we do not have to rely so much on our ability to follow vague advice to eat small portions, eat a lot of fruit and vegetables, and avoid foods that are high in fat and sugar. We do not need to stress about specific foods if we focus on the numbers. Nutrition should not be a guessing game.

We are designed to grab calories whenever they are available. We are designed to reward ourselves when something tastes good. In a time where half of the US population is overweight, why are we left with these vague guidelines from which we are supposed to shape our entire diets? A much more effective approach is to have numeric guidelines to follow. It is much more difficult to measure our adherence to subjective, vague guidelines.

Of course, you can adjust your tracking technique to fit your goals and preferences. Many of us do not need to worry about hitting exact numbers every day, but by approximately reaching our daily goals for macronutrient intake, we can get on the right track. Once you see what portion sizes look like and practice weighing and tracking food, you can phase out of tracking exact measurements if you would rather not weigh your food. However, weighing food and gaining an understanding of portion sizes is necessary in the beginning stages of flexible dieting. "Winging it" is not considered a superior approach for anything that matters in life, and it should not be considered a superior approach for tracking one's dietary intake.

## Weighing Food

You have calculated your macros and have all these food ideas floating in your head. So now what? The next step comes from the fact that portion size is critical to successful flexible dieting. Your usual dinner at your favorite restaurant might be well over your dietary fat goals for the day, but if you eat half of it or ask to make a simple substitution, it might work out just fine.

For all meals that you make yourself, a food scale is a wise investment. Try to measure rice using a measuring cup and you can easily see how much variation there can be depending on how many grains you scoop into the cup. Weighing food to find its actual weight is crucial to maintaining accuracy when tracking macronutrients. Once you start weighing food, you will quickly notice just how inaccurate nutrition labels and food databases can be. A slice of bread might be listed as 30 g on the label, but you weigh it out and find it is 38 g (simply multiply by 1.267 to track it in this case). To increase accuracy, never measure foods by volume; measure by weight.

Even when we measure food by weight, we must deal with inconsistencies. For example, the amount of water in and around cooked rice could affect the reading. Weigh your food carefully to avoid any common mistakes. Set the scale to zero before placing the food on the scale. Be careful not to include any dishes or utensils in your weight measurement. Pay attention to whether the nutrition data (e.g. nutrition label) is referring to the food in its cooked or raw form.

While you need to be careful, you do not need to change your normal routine as much as you might think. Many people think that they will have to prepare only single-serving portions of their food when they start weighing and tracking food, but that is not the case. You can cook an entire recipe, calculate the calorie and macronutrient composition for the entire dish, and simply divide by the number of portions. If you are going to be the only one eating the recipe, then this will lead to no error. Let's say you get a portion of turkey chili with a ton of beans and not a lot of turkey for one meal, but you eat the entire recipe's yield by the end of the week. Or let's say you made banana bread and cut some pieces larger than others, but you eat all the pieces. By the end of the week, the average serving of chili or banana bread was the serving size you intended for, so all is good. If other people will also eat the recipe, you can either measure everything for single-serving sizes or just estimate. The latter approach can lead to slight inaccuracies. It just depends on how exact you want to be.

## Getting into a Routine

Part of what makes flexible dieting so enticing is the idea that you can eat whatever you want, but this freedom should not be mistaken for carelessness. You might find that you prefer to plan your days in advance instead of tracking on the spot. You can track with an app, like MyFitnessPal, in a spreadsheet or word document, or with a pencil and paper. Whichever way you do it, once you get the hang of it, tracking will become a normal part of your daily routine that requires very little thought and time. Here are some tips as you get started:

1.  Come up with some go-to meals in case you do not have time to think of something fancy. Planning can help you avoid grabbing something low in nutrients and high in calories, which you might regret after the fact, especially when you realize your meal was not as filling as it could have been.

2. Because protein is the most satiating macronutrient, it can help to have protein as the focal point of each meal. Once you have a protein source, add some plants and, if needed, extra fat (some protein sources already have a significant amount of fat), and you're good to go.

3. When you first start tracking your intake, aim for balance in each meal. Get into the habit of incorporating whole foods and plenty of nutrients so that you do not have to track micronutrients every single day. Note that flexible dieting might seem difficult and confusing at first. There is a learning curve, but it will get easier. Just like anything else, it might be awkward or even scary at first, but once flexible dieting is part of your everyday routine, it becomes nearly automatic.

4. If you find yourself really struggling, try to keep your goals at the forefront of your mind. When you are confronted with a difficult choice and want to go off track, visualize what you want to achieve. Envision your future self. What do you look like? Where are you? What are you doing? Try to imagine every detail, even colors. Now do what you know you need to do to get there.

## Meal Planning

Part of the allure of flexible dieting is that you do not have to prepare your meals ahead of time. However, as we have mentioned already, meal planning can be a key step in sticking to nutrient intake goals. For many of us, it can be annoying to calculate the macronutrient intake of a meal each time we want to eat and then subtract that from our daily goal. (For others of us, it can be fun.)

We are more likely to eat something if it is convenient. If you have trouble sticking to your diet, a simple trick is to make nutrient-dense, "macro-friendly" foods more accessible and make calorie-dense, low-nutrient foods less accessible. What exactly does this mean? Make sure lean protein sources are cooked and ready to go. Have fibrous vegetables, fruit, whole grains, and low-fat dairy on deck and ready to make a meal. If the meals are already made and ready to be eaten, we are simply more likely to reach for them. Minimally processed foods, like precut vegetables, can be extremely useful, and if you do not want to cook meals yourself, there are many services that sell prepackaged, nutrient-dense meals that display grams of protein, carbohydrates, and fat right on the container. If you would rather spend some money than time on having meals ready, it might be worth doing some research to see if there are any services in your area or if you could locate one that ships to your location. There are also cheaper options, like microwaveable meals, which are often diet-friendly and always have nutrition facts listed on the labels.

When making sure nutrient-dense foods are readily accessible, we should also make nutrient-poor foods less accessible to us. Often this means simply not buying them. If you are someone who accounts for one cookie in your daily macronutrient goals but then reaches for one or two more, you might be better off simply not having them around. If you want a treat, you can go out and buy just one.

The first step to meal planning is to decide how many meals per day you want to consume. As we will see in the "Meal Timing" chapter, this depends on what works best for your preferences and schedule. There is no magic number of meals to help you reach your goals. For our example, we will use five meals. While you will probably want to adjust the composition of each meal depending on factors like workout timing and personal preference, for convenience we will divide a sample daily macronutrient intake into five even meals. If we use a daily target of 50 g fat, 250 g carbohydrates, and 150 g protein, then each meal comes to 10 g fat, 50 g carbs, and 30 g protein per meal.

Once you have the macronutrient content of a single meal, an easy way to plan the meal is to start with a protein source. For this example, let's choose egg whites. In 243 g of egg whites, there are 2 g carbohydrates, 26 g protein, and virtually no fat. Next, choose a carbohydrate source. An easy way to ensure high nutrient content is to choose a vegetable or fruit and a starch. For this example, we'll choose spinach and shredded potatoes. In 30 g of spinach, there are approximately 1 g carbohydrates, 1 g protein, and virtually no fat. In 250 g of potato, there are 43 g carbohydrates, 5 g protein, and virtually no fat. Now let's choose a fat source. We could choose an oil to cook it in, but since we are already using egg whites, let's add two whole eggs for fat. That adds 10 g of fat, 2 g of carbs, and 12 g of protein. So we can decrease the egg whites to half the serving size we had before to yield 13 g of protein from egg whites. Our grand total has 10 g of fat, 47 g of carbohydrates, and 30 g of protein. Then we can add a squirt of ketchup or grab a few blueberries for the extra 3 g of carbohydrates or carry them over in our dietary budget for use in another meal.

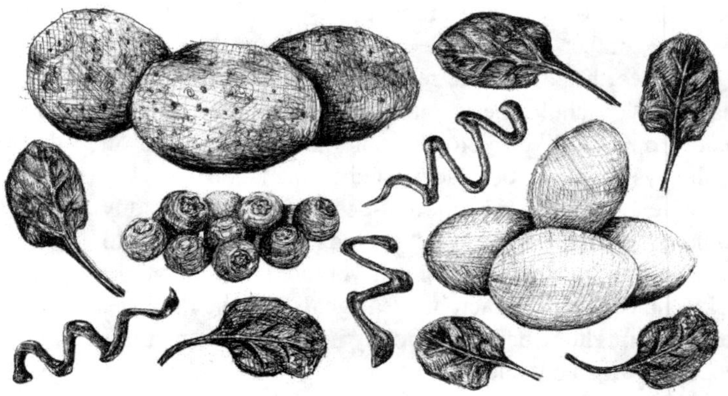

Once you have some go-to food or meal options, it is up to you whether you want to continue meal planning while flexible dieting. Even if you do not plan days or meals in advance, you may want to have some "macro-friendly" meals in mind that you can resort to in a pinch. "Macro-friendly" refers to a food or meal that you can easily fit into your daily intake. For most of us, a macro-friendly option is high in protein and low in fat, carbohydrates, or both. If you frequently go to Starbucks, for example, it can help to identify a few menu options that you know you can easily fit into your daily macronutrient guidelines. At the back of this book is a table of macro-friendly options at some popular restaurants. Menus change all the time, so be sure to consult the most updated nutrition data available for the restaurant of interest.

## Everything Counts

A common mistake when someone starts tracking his or her intake is to forget to track everything. It sounds like a simple concept, but unless you are used to tracking everything you eat or generally obsessing over food, accounting for every morsel of food might not come naturally. Food is typically not thought of as something for which we have to budget. Unfortunately, we have evolved to desire food that is high in fat or sugar whenever it is available to us, and today in the US these types of foods are extremely accessible to many of us. But even in this time where foods are manufactured to be tasty and cheap, it is possible to maintain a balanced diet that is conducive to overall health and fitness goals.

To maximize success with flexible dieting, we need to track

everything that enters our mouths, including: gum, mints, artificial sweetener packets, pre-workout supplements, fish oil supplements, cooking sprays, those bites we take when cooking dinner or packing lunch, our morning coffee, and everything else that we consume. Foods under five calories per serving are allowed to be labeled as "calorie free." One or a few of these foods per day will not add much to your overall intake, but these can add up if you use twenty sprays, scoops, or packets of something per day. And yes, vegetables must be tracked. No food is a freebie. Vegetables are a nutrient-dense source of carbohydrates (especially fiber) that also contain protein and even fat. There are no magic foods that you do not need to track. All foods or beverages that provide us with energy must be accounted for.

An exception to this rule can be when you take the same supplement or add a packet of artificial sweetener to your breakfast every day—for example, if you take two of the same brand fish oil capsules every single day but never track it. In this example, you will always think your dietary fat intake is about 2 g lower than it is. Other than that, there is no harm done. This is a systematic error. Similarly, if you eat one cup of spinach every single day and never track it, the only loss is not having those nutrients and calories added into your daily totals. But because it is the same mistake every single day, this miscalculation would not explain any weight fluctuations or changes in progress. The downfall of this way of thinking is that we have off days, we take vacations, and we change our routines. Since many of us do not have habits that we maintain every single day of our lives, it is wise to use the "everything counts" approach to optimize progress.

If you forget to track something that is not a typical part of your daily routine, like taking a bite of food that you are cooking for a family dinner, it can lead to inconsistent tracking over time, since you will not be sampling the same size of the same food every day. If you sneak a few bites of cookie dough today, but tomorrow nothing is unaccounted for, and the next day after that you take a few bites of the family dinner while it is cooking, and the following day you give half of one of your meals to your dog, you can see how the pattern is inconsistent. This is random error, and the way to avoid it is, as we mentioned, to track everything that enters your mouth—nothing more and nothing less.

For many of us, tracking everything we eat requires practice. If you ever mindlessly grab a bite of something to eat without realizing it, try writing down everything you eat in a day and see if it helps. If you miss anything, keep trying until you master the process. Developing mindfulness about eating is a prerequisite to flexible dieting. No meal, snack, or drink should go without notice or thought. One method for improving this awareness is to avoid multitasking. As the Zen saying goes, "When you drink, just drink. When you walk, just walk."

If you don't have a specific deadline for your goal, if you are susceptible to an unhealthy obsession with food, or if you just want to prioritize flexibility, then you do not need to be as much of a stickler for tracking everything. But if your goal is specific, for example, to achieve a certain percent body fat or body weight by a certain date, then it is critical to make sure you track everything that you consume.

## Ask Questions

Getting started with flexible dieting involves a basic understanding of food and its nutrients and how they can affect your body, but it also requires a willingness to learn more and ask questions when you need more information about the contents of a meal or about whether the meal can fit into your diet for the day.

Do not be afraid to ask about the ingredients of a meal if they are not listed or to request a substitute or an omission from a meal. A regular hamburger can become a low-carb, high-protein meal if you forgo the bun and switch out fries for a salad (dressing on the side). Grilled chicken, vegetables, and potato might sound like an easy-to-track meal until you find out everything is dripping in butter, but a simple request to omit any oil or butter can make this a low-fat meal option.

Once you know what kind of meal you need to fit your macronutrient intake goals, it becomes easy to find meals that fit your guidelines if you know the ingredients. Unfortunately, individuals who are not educated about nutrition tend to be labeled as more easygoing since they never ask questions about the food. People who care about their health and well-being are labeled as picky eaters or even a nuisance. But when you find the courage to ask questions, people will notice your confidence and purpose and perhaps even become curious. Your passion to better yourself can be contagious.

We may even be fooled by the names of meals themselves. As we saw earlier, a grilled chicken salad can be full of fat, sugar, and sodium. Unfortunately, preying on the health-conscious seems to be a marketing tactic. But just because you see a lean protein source or "salad" in the name of a meal does not necessarily mean it is a safe choice. The good news is that you can often figure out the actual nutrient composition of a meal by simply looking up the nutrition data, which is usually accessible through the websites of chain restaurants or by asking questions.

Take, for example, "Chicken and Shrimp Carbonara." If you don't know what carbonara is, and even if you do, it sounds like this could be a macro-friendly option. The Chicken and Shrimp Carbonara at Olive Garden has 114 g fat (61 g saturated fat), 78 g carbohydrates, and 66 g protein. I knew that a spaghetti dish would have a decent amount of carbohydrates, but I was astounded when I first read these nutrition facts. Where was the fat coming from? The recipe for carbonara includes whole eggs, cheese, and bacon: three sources of fat. These are accompanied by butter, lard, oil, sometimes cream, or some combination of these. This Italian dish could still be a decent choice if it were served in a reasonable portion size, but when we combine these ingredients with American chain-restaurant-sized portions, it is clear why the fat content and overall calorie content of the dish are so high.

Facts about nutrition can be wrongly conveyed through marketing tactics, the media, and even health professionals. While it is wise to do your own research and to learn about nutrition, watch out for wrongly interpreted data, sensationalized media reports, and myths. As a science, nutrition starts with the research. However, as food is always a hot topic, associations shown in research studies are often misinterpreted and then blown up in news headlines. For topics that lack a sufficient quantity of research literature, we like to make up our own explanations and theories. Be careful about the source of your nutrition news. Think critically. Although each of us has his or her own metabolic needs and may or may not have major health diagnoses that affect specific dietary needs, we are all human. Food and its marketing affect us in predictable, verifiable ways.

Nutrition is also largely absent from our children's education. In physics, we often do not connect the dots between thermodynamics and energy balance in our everyday life. In chemistry, we usually do not learn about macronutrients. In biology, we rarely go into detail about nutrient absorption after digestion occurs. We all eventually specialize in a specific field, and most of us never learn about nutrition in detail, yet many of us think we are experts. Unfortunately, eating food does not make us experts in nutrition.

## The Potato Paradox

Keep in mind that even if you prepare all your food yourself, the available data does not accurately reflect the specific foods that you have. You can look up the data for a medium potato, and once you get past the first hurdle (how many grams does a medium potato weigh?), you will find that there are several possible options for calorie, carbohydrate, and sugar contents for the same exact size potato. This is what I refer to as "the potato paradox."

The first layer of confusion comes from the type of potato. You might think that there are white potatoes and sweet potatoes, but all white potatoes are not equal, and all sweet potatoes are not equal. Generally, white potatoes have a higher glycemic index, but sweet potatoes have a higher simple sugar content. There are different types of sweet potatoes though. You may have seen orange, white, or purple ones. Each can have a different sugar, fiber, and overall nutrient content.

Beyond the type of potato lie several other factors: individual potato genetic makeup, methods of storage and cooking, and temperature are just a few of these factors. One potato might have thicker skin (and therefore more fiber) or more sugar. Cooking the potato makes it easier to digest, but allowing the cooked potato to cool down makes it more resistant to digestion. The glycemic index of a cooled, cooked potato is therefore lower than a potato fresh out of the oven. The specific cooking method can also change the nutrient content, even if you do not add any extra ingredients. Baking a whole potato is different than cutting it into little pieces and baking them into crunchier fries or chips. Even though the only ingredient in either case is a potato, the baked whole potato will have much more water, and therefore fewer calories, per the same weight serving size.

This applies to all foods, not just potatoes. Unless your kitchen is also a laboratory, it is unlikely that you will be able to measure with a high degree of accuracy. But that does not mean that you should not try! It is better to be 95% on point, or even 80%, than 50% or 0%.

## How Accurate Do I Need to Be?

It is important to be as exact as possible with your measurements. In general, the more accurate you are, the better your results will be. Keep in mind that the total daily food intake is much more important than the timing or composition of any one meal. If one meal is off track, you can make it up at the next meal consistent with your dietary budget. While it is a good idea to consume balanced meals and to prioritize carbohydrates before a workout and protein after a workout, you can still progress just fine if you do not follow meal timing guidelines.

The point of tracking to the exact gram is to have consistency, but foods are not consistent. Because food nutrition information will often not match what has been advertised or publicized, aiming for daily macronutrient target ranges of 5–10 g or more depending on what works for you can be enough to stay on track. Some people prefer to aim for the exact number every day.

Nutrition labels can be misleading. The following information comes from the FDA website: Calorie values less than 5 can be expressed as 0. Calorie values less than or equal to 50 can be rounded to the nearest 5 calorie increment. Calorie values higher than 50 can be rounded to the nearest 10 calorie increment. Grams of fat greater than or equal to 5 can be rounded to the nearest 1 g increment. Grams of carbohydrates and protein greater than or equal to 1 can also be rounded to the nearest 1 g increment.

Calorie content on nutrition labels can use specific Atwater factors listed in table 13 of USDA Handbook No. 74, which was revised in 1973 or general factors of 4, 4, and 9 calories per gram for carbohydrates, protein, and fat, respectively. In the USDA table referenced, the factor to be applied for ingested protein from eggs is 4.36 calories per gram. The factor to be applied for ingested protein from 100% wheat bran is 1.82. You can see how different these values are from each other but also from the generic value of 4.

Class I nutrients, or those added in fortified or fabricated foods, must be present at 100% or more of the value that appears on the label. Class II nutrients, vitamins, minerals, protein, total carbohydrate, dietary fiber, other carbohydrate, polyunsaturated and monounsaturated fat, or potassium that occur naturally in a food product must be present at 80% or more of the value that appears on the label. Third Group nutrients, which include calories, sugars, total fat, saturated fat, cholesterol, and sodium, must be present at 120% or less of the value that appears on the label.

Food databases estimate values even further. It is impractical to perform chemical analyses on all foods in a database. According to a 1996 article by Schakel, Buzzard, and Gebhardt, appropriate procedures for estimating such values include simply using values from a similar food; calculating values for a different form of the same food, that is, calculating values for a cooked or processed form of a food using its raw values; calculating values for a whole food based on data for its parts; and by adding known values for ingredients in a recipe. These are methods that you can use yourself if nutrition data is not readily available for a specific food.

Tracking might seem like an impossible task. There will always be factors that are out of your control. Just as we can't always control our body's internal bodyweight regulation system, we can't always control the accuracy of the data that we track. But by maximizing accuracy for the things we can control, we can optimize our results. Weigh food when you can, estimate when you can't, and always prioritize nutrient-dense foods.

In addition to nutrition data inaccuracies, we are not living in a laboratory. Each day, we have a different energy expenditure. The good news is that it doesn't really matter since the average is more important than any single meal or day. At the same time, if you find that your energy expenditure varies substantially from day to day, you might benefit from carb cycling, i.e. having "high-carb" and "low-carb" days, or otherwise redistributing your macronutrients across the week. If you have extremely intense or long workouts, or if you find that you simply prefer to eat more on certain days and less on others, then this might be a good approach for you.

While flexible dieting allows us to fit any type of food into our diet, it is not an excuse to eat whatever we want and to "make it fit" by adjusting our macros for the rest of the week. Whatever way you choose to apply (or not apply) flexible dieting to your life, do it with care, and do it with intention. As Roald Dahl once said, "Lukewarm is no good."

# 6
# MICRONUTRIENTS

As difficult as it is to get accurate data for macronutrients, it is even more difficult to get accurate data for micronutrients. Unfortunately, whole foods, which typically contain the largest amounts of micronutrients per serving, cannot each be individually lab tested. While many processed foods are meant to be as close to identical as possible, each piece of produce is unique. For this reason, your best bet is to focus on diet variety when it comes to micronutrients. Tracking individual micronutrients will take up time with little reward since factors like ripeness, cooking method, and temperature can affect the micronutrient content of food.

Although it takes time, it is still possible to track your intake of individual micronutrients. The proportion of micronutrients remaining after cooking a food is called the retention factor. If you know the amount of a specific nutrient in a serving of raw food, you can multiply by the retention factor to find out how much of that nutrient will be left in your serving after cooking. You can do this for each micronutrient and end up with approximate values that will give a estimation of your daily micronutrient intake. But most of us who consume a balanced diet and do not have major health symptoms or diagnoses can forgo this level of tracking.

In addition to the difficulty of obtaining micronutrient data that accurately represent what we are consuming, it can be difficult to determine how much of each micronutrient each of us needs. The Institute of Medicine (IOM) has set forth recommendations called the dietary reference intakes (DRI). These reference values include the Recommended Dietary Allowance (RDA), Estimated Average Requirement (EAR), Adequate Intake (AI), and Tolerable Upper Intake Level (UL). The Acceptable Macronutrient Distribution Ranges (AMDR) for macronutrients mentioned earlier are also part of the DRI. The RDA is considered sufficient to meet the needs of 97.5% of healthy individuals of a specific gender and age group, while the EAR is considered sufficient to meet the needs of only 50% of individuals in a specific group. The RDA is estimated to be about 20% greater than the EAR. When there is no RDA available due to insufficient data, a micronutrient will have an AI, which is an estimate of what would meet the needs of a population. The UL is the highest amount that is considered safe (without side effects) for 97.5% of a group. In addition to these different requirements for different genders and age groups, certain populations, like athletes, menstruating females, or unhealthy individuals, may have different requirements for certain nutrients than a typical individual. Most of us can get by with less than the RDA requirements, so when we use the RDA as a guideline, we are playing it safe.

Vitamins are typically classified as fat soluble or water soluble. Fat-soluble vitamins are absorbed in the lymph and stored in the liver or adipose tissue. If we don't consume enough dietary fat, we cannot properly absorb fat-soluble vitamins. Water-soluble vitamins are not stored in the body in very high quantities, and excess amounts are excreted through urine.

Minerals are necessary for normal body functions and can be categorized by the amount of each that we require. Macrominerals are those that we require in larger amounts, and trace elements, or microminerals, are those that we require in smaller amounts. Minerals are consumed in their ion states.

Vitamins and minerals do not encompass all micronutrients. Phytonutrients, or phytochemicals, are naturally occurring compounds found in plants that contribute to an abundance of health benefits in humans. There is much we still do not know about phytonutrients. A diet rich in whole, plant-based foods is critical for ensuring that we take advantage of their benefits. It is largely unknown whether supplements containing phytonutrients have the same benefits of foods containing phytonutrients.

In addition to micronutrients, there are microorganisms found in and on food, as well as around us in other ways, that are beneficial to our health. A large portion of our microbiomes live in our large intestine, so the food we consume has a substantial impact on the kinds of bacteria that live in our bodies.

Probiotics are microorganisms such as live bacteria and yeasts that have beneficial qualities. Probiotics can change or repopulate bacteria in our gastrointestinal (GI) tract to improve GI health. Fermented dairy products like yogurt, kefir, and aged cheeses are sources of probiotics. Nondairy probiotic sources include sauerkraut, kimchi, miso, tempeh, cultured nondairy yogurts, and kombucha.

Prebiotics are nondigestible food components, like inulin and galactooligosaccharides, that promote the growth or activity of microorganisms. Gum arabic, chicory root, artichoke, dandelion greens, garlic, and leeks contain high quantities of prebiotic fiber. Onions, asparagus, wheat bran, whole-wheat flour, and bananas are also good sources of prebiotic fiber.

## Common Deficiencies

Tracking micronutrients and microorganisms might be overkill, but it is a good idea to either get lab work done before starting a diet to see if you have deficiencies or to track your intake of all micronutrients for a few days to a week to get an idea of your current intake.

Conservative estimates suggest that over 25% of the world population is deficient in iron, with even higher percentages of children, menstruating and pregnant women, and vegetarians and vegans being deficient. Fatigue, weakness, brain fog, and a weakened immune system can result from iron deficiency. Iron deficiency can also lead to anemia in which blood's ability to carry oxygen throughout the body is decreased due to a deficiency in red blood cells or hemoglobin. To get your iron fix, enjoy a serving of liver, shellfish, or red meat. If you do not like any of those, beans and seeds are excellent plant sources.

Data suggest that nearly half of US adults may be deficient in vitamin D. Vitamin D deficiency can be difficult to detect due to a lack of noticeable symptoms. Vitamin D deficiency can go unnoticed until muscle weakness or bone loss starts to occur. Vitamin D deficiency can cause growth delays in children and decreased bone density in people of all ages. Fatty fish is high in vitamin D, and vegetarians can get high doses in egg yolks. Vegans will need to work harder, but keep in mind that we also produce vitamin D when we are exposed to the sun.

Like vitamin D, vitamin B12 can be difficult to obtain from diet alone, particularly for vegans and many vegetarians. Vitamin B12 helps make DNA and keep nerve and blood cells healthy. Shellfish, organ meat, and other meat contain the highest doses of vitamin B12, while dairy and eggs are good vegetarian sources. Plant sources include nori seaweed, tempeh, and dirt found on produce.

The iodization of salt has greatly decreased iodine deficiency across the globe in recent years. Iodine deficiency can cause an enlarged thyroid, a condition called goiter, which can cause weight gain, among other symptoms. Iodine deficiency can also cause developmental abnormalities in infants and young children. Iodine is found in the soil and sea, so high doses are available in seaweed, fish, dairy, and iodized salt. People who are trying to be health conscious by switching to non-iodized specialty salts might be missing out on the benefits of iodized salt.

Data suggest that certain populations such as adolescent females and women over fifty years of age are not meeting calcium intake requirements. The body will take calcium from bones if we do not get enough from food, so low calcium intake puts us at risk of decreased bone density and osteoporosis. Boned fish and dairy are excellent sources of calcium. Dark green vegetables can be a good source of calcium, but note that large portions are needed to get the same amount of calcium that we can easily get from boned fish and dairy.

These are just some common micronutrient deficiencies. Many of us are also deficient in magnesium, potassium, or both, while vitamin A deficiency is a huge problem in some other parts of the world.

For many vitamins and minerals, populations most at risk for deficiencies are the elderly, athletes, low-income populations, and individuals with health conditions that prevent the absorption of certain nutrients. Nevertheless, it is possible for healthy individuals to be deficient in one or more micronutrients. If you do not consume whole foods from all food groups, it can be difficult to get enough of all micronutrients. Consuming a balanced, varied diet is the best way to ensure adequate nutrient intake.

## Fortification

According to the World Health Organization (WHO) and Food and Agricultural Organization (FAO), fortification is the process of "deliberately increasing the content of an essential micronutrient" in a food, whereas enrichment refers to a type of fortification in which micronutrient content is increased to make up for what was lost during processing.

Even though fortification often uses synthetic vitamins and minerals, the increase in nutrient content of foods has almost eliminated the deficiency of several vitamins in America and other developed countries. The synthetic vitamins used for fortification are usually easily absorbed, but there are some exceptions. For instance, drinking skim milk fortified with vitamin A and D can increase our intake of these vitamins, but since they are fat soluble, we will not optimally absorb them unless we eat something else that contains fat. As with most potential issues stemming from single foods, however, these problems can be solved by ensuring that our diets are high in variety.

Fortification has been a remarkable public health intervention and an overwhelming excuse to fill our diets with foods that would otherwise be poor choices, like sugary cereal and snacks. Imagine what would happen if sugary sodas and potato chips were fortified and advertised for their new and improved nutrient content. Unfortunately, the macronutrient composition of these foods would have to dramatically change for these foods to merit a larger role in our diets.

The advantage of whole foods over fortified foods does not come entirely from vitamins and minerals but also from other beneficial compounds, like phytonutrients. People whose diets are rich in fortified foods might get more vitamins and minerals than if they were to eat only whole foods, but they are missing out on other beneficial nutrients that cannot now be obtained from fortified foods.

## Variety is Key

McCollum and Davis's single-grain experiment in the early 1900s was one of the first instances to show that macronutrient composition is not the only aspect to consider when it comes to consuming a healthy diet. In their experiment, cows were fed diets consisting of a single grain. The outcome was that cows fed a diet of only corn or only bran were healthy, but cows fed a diet of only wheat were unhealthy. It turns out that the cows on the wheat diet were suffering from vitamin A deficiency. This illustrated the importance of nutrients other than macronutrients in our diets and the negative impact of a restrictive diet.

Appearance and performance are good indicators of progress, but you can still be on track and hiding a nutrient deficiency or potentially serious health diagnosis. Always put your long-term health first; it is what allows you to meet your short-term goals. A varied diet rich in whole foods will help to ensure adequate intake of micronutrients.

# 7

# WHAT TO EAT

The accepted approach to flexible dieting is that you are free to choose which foods you want to eat to meet macronutrient goals; however, a diet that is conducive to fat loss and/or muscle growth is one that is high in nutrient-dense foods. As we have discussed, micronutrients play critical roles in essential body functions. Inadequate intake of vitamins and minerals can not only hinder progress but also negatively impact upon overall health. However, if the foundation of your diet is varied and consists of nutrient-dense foods, having a few treats here and there can be justified if you are still able to reach your daily macronutrient goals.

## Quantity versus Quality

The foundation of flexible dieting is built on the fact that quantity of food consumed is more important than the quality. A healthy body weight and composition are protective against poor metabolic outcomes and diseases. It is always better to consume appropriate portions. Even if quality is excellent, food in the wrong quantities can be detrimental. Overeating organic, nutrient-dense, omega-3-fortified, sugar-free, natural foods is still overeating! You cannot trick your body into altering the fact that energy balance is an equation. If intake is higher than expenditure, you will gain weight. If intake is lower than expenditure, you will lose weight. As mentioned in the beginning of this book, internal regulation of energy balance is complex, while external regulation of energy balance is much simpler; external regulation of energy balance is largely influenced by the amount of food we eat and the amount of activity we perform.

There are many claims that diet quality is more important than quantity; the rationale comes from the fact that it is easier to consume appropriate portions of nutrient-dense foods than nutrient-poor, calorie-dense food. It is easy to consume excess calories in the form of potato chips or sugar-sweetened beverages. It is much more difficult to consume excess calories in the form of fruit and vegetables. Just ask someone with a habit of drinking sugar-sweetened soda to add up how many calories the person consumes from soda each day. Then ask someone with a habit of eating fruit and vegetables to add up how many calories he or she consumes from fruit and vegetables each day. Calories from drinking sugar add up much faster than calories from chewing solid boluses of fiber, sugar, and other nutrients.

When the entire caloric intake is greater than expenditure, weight gain occurs. It is simply easier to tilt the scale with "low-quality" foods. These include foods that are high in sugar, fat, or both but low in protein, fiber, and volume. In other words, they are high in calories without being very filling.

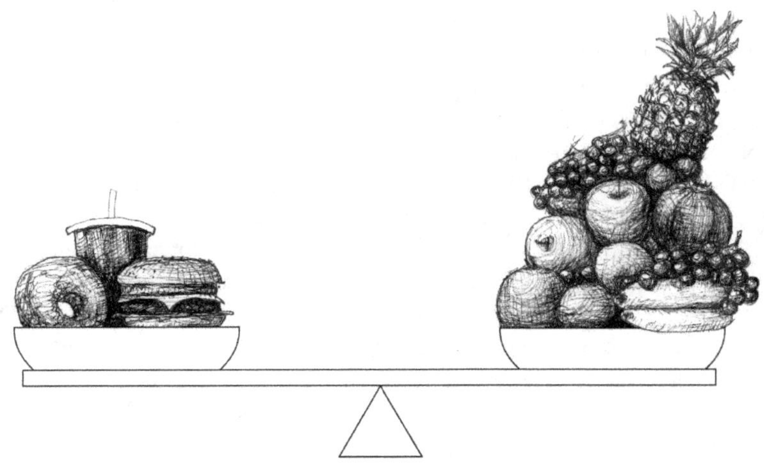

However, claims that specific foods can slow down your metabolism or otherwise cause weight gain are largely unfounded. Total metabolism can be influenced by factors like age, height, weight, hormone levels, physical activity level, but not single foods. Weight gain is caused by eating a caloric surplus regardless of the food being consumed, so unless you typically consume enough of one food to exceed the total daily caloric intake required to maintain your weight (e.g. drinking liters of soda or large bags of potato chips per day), then a specific food is not the source of weight gain. You can drink a small sugary soda or eat a small bag of potato chips every day and maintain or even lose weight just depending on how your total caloric intake stacks up against your total expenditure.

It is true that certain foods are more likely to promote weight gain, but it is not the foods themselves that cause the weight gain. Remember the difference between correlation and causation. The consumption of a particular food itself does not cause the outcome. For example, people who consume sugary soda might be more likely to develop obesity. This does not mean that soda itself causes obesity. It likely means that people who consume sugary soda are more likely to consume an excess of calories, which can lead to obesity over time.

It is even more difficult to research the effects of specific nutrients on humans, as we cannot entirely eliminate a nutrient from individuals' diets to create a comparison group of subjects. Often, we are left with results that indicate associations or correlations, but not causations. These results are then misinterpreted and sensationalized.

## The "Superfood" Conundrum

As we have previously touched on, there are truly no "good" or "bad" foods but rather more or less nutritious foods. Does that mean certain foods are better than others? What about "superfoods" that supposedly prevent or cure disease, burn belly fat, or increase brain function?

Clearly, no one food by itself can accomplish any of these feats, although a diet that is rich in nutritious foods can improve overall health and protect against certain diseases. Specific claims like burning belly fat or increasing brain function often come from studies that indicate a small association that is sensationalized by the media. Can a food burn belly fat? No. A study might have found an association with fat loss, but simply eating a food or taking a supplement or adding a spice will not burn belly fat. Burning fat means that the body loses fat and oxygen in the form of carbon dioxide and water via breath and sweat. You can increase this process by moving more and eating less. Brain function is also a result of "exercising" your brain. Intelligence is supposedly about 50% heritable, while the other 50% depends on environment. Most of the second 50% involves thinking and doing activities to strengthen connections between neurons—not eating a handful of magic foods. While specific foods can indeed have a small association with positive outcomes, superfoods are not as "super" as they are often advertised to be.

The real trick behind superfoods and other dietary products with extraordinary health claims is that they are often sold in bulk in the form of powders and pills marketed as supplements as opposed to foods. If the point of consuming these foods was to fill your diet with nutritious, whole foods, then why are we purchasing them in the form of processed supplements?

Real "superfoods" should include both foods that are high in nutrients and foods that make us feel good, even happy. A flexible dieting approach encourages eating for both physical and mental health. To the extent that any food can be characterized as a superfood, I would consider spinach to be one because of its high nutrient density. Spinach is high in vitamin K, vitamin A, fiber, and many other nutrients, yet low in calories.

At the same time, homemade cookies might also deserve to be considered a superfood for their mental health benefits. There are few things in life that make me happier than a fresh, homemade cookie with a crunchy exterior and a chewy, melted inside. The typical cookie recipe yields a product that is low in vitamins, minerals, and protein and high in fat and sugar, but the experience of eating one makes me happy, especially when I know the batch was made with love. Flexible dieting allows room for both types of superfoods. A diet that is low in nutrients is no good, but a diet that prevents you from enjoying the texture and taste of foods is also no good.

Sure, there are foods that give you more "bang for your buck" when it comes to nutrient density. Salmon is high in omega-3 fatty acids, protein, and vitamins and minerals. Kale is full of vitamin A, vitamin C, vitamin K, fiber, and nonnutritive compounds, and kale is also lower than spinach in oxalates, which can bind and prevent the absorption of calcium. Beef liver is one of the most nutrient-dense foods you can eat. The list goes on.

However, we cannot simply eat these nutrient-dense foods and expect to see progress! To reach both short-term and long-term health goals, we must consider calories, macronutrients, and micronutrients. At the same time, a truly holistic approach through flexible dieting requires that we balance our ability to make smart food choices with our unique preferences and overall happiness.

## The Power of Whole Foods

Which foods are conducive to maintaining or improving physical health? Among the most obvious foods are the ones that are consistent with the USDA MyPlate; these are the foods that many of us recognize as "healthy" options: whole grains, lean protein, fruit, vegetables, nuts, legumes, and low-fat dairy. But it is easy to see how misinformed and confused many of us are even by starting with these. Some people may choose to avoid dairy, legumes, grains, and sugar, for example, so what are the best options? What makes us healthy?

Whole foods are highly nutritious, and many processed foods are highly nutritious. The USDA MyPlate shows no place for foods low in nutrients. What about Pop-Tarts? Those are not whole grains. Classic, all-American foods are nowhere to be found on the plate. Are french fries a vegetable? Does orange juice count as a fruit? Where's the pizza? Even foods that are low in nutrients provide us with energy.

In terms of nutrition, "better" food choices are simply those with high nutrient density. Any food that is satiating and full of vitamins and minerals yet low in calories would be an example of this. Lean fish is leaner than hamburger meat. Quinoa is higher in fiber and vitamins and minerals than a bun. If we look at 200-calorie portions for all four of these foods, they each have different macronutrient compositions. They are unequal in terms of everything except calories.

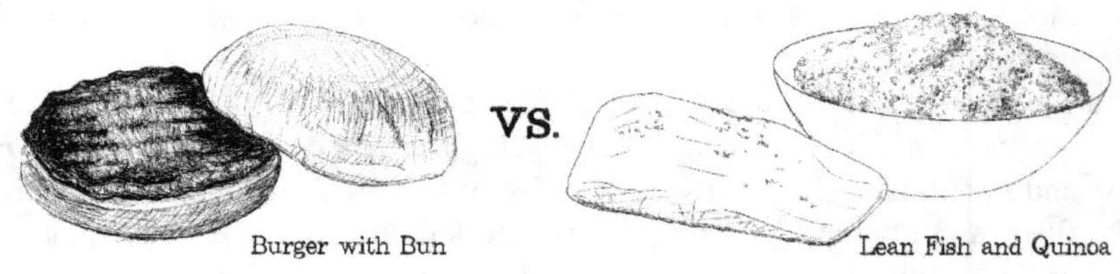


In 3 oz of 80% lean ground beef there are 14 g fat and 20 g protein, while 6 oz cod has 6 g fat and 36 g protein. A hamburger bun and 1 cup of quinoa both have approximately 4 g fat, 35 g carbohydrates, and 7 g protein, but quinoa has twice as much fiber and 58% of your daily value (% DV) manganese, 30% DV magnesium, 28% DV phosphorus, 19% folate, and many other key nutrients that a bun does not have.

Foods that provide us with the same amount of energy and make the same deposit in our personal macronutrient bank for the day do not necessarily supply us with the same amounts of vitamins or minerals. We can imagine that if we ate the less nutritious choices for all meals, we would end up low in certain vitamins and minerals. We can still make poor food choices and reach our macronutrient intake goals every day. What matters is the overall dietary intake pattern, not the composition of a single meal.

Many people consume a thousand or more meals in a year. One meal that has too much or too little of anything will not have a significant impact on overall health; however, consistently choosing too much or too little can make a difference in health and well-being even if you do not notice a difference in body weight or appearance.

Although whole foods are praised for their high nutrient content, there may be more to their benefits than specific nutrients alone. Whole foods have been shown to have a more favorable impact on disease risk factors than supplementation of nutrients found in those foods. It is unclear whether there is some form of the Gestalt principle at play in nature, that is, the whole is greater than the sum of its parts. In any case, we know that getting our nutrients from food typically has more benefits than getting them from supplements.

While whole foods certainly are nutrient-dense, health-promoting options, classifying certain foods as "clean" or "good" and others as "bad" is not a healthy way of implementing flexible dieting. This way of thinking is often a gateway to negative thoughts and obsessions about food. If you want to avoid certain foods for personal reasons, go ahead, but there is no reason to avoid any one food for health reasons if there is no underlying health diagnosis or intolerance to consider.

Foods do not have magic properties that make them either good or bad for losing or gaining weight. Calories are king, so if you really mess up and eat way too much fat or cannot get enough fat, for example, don't stress. Just do the math and hit your overall calories for the day.

## Dieting versus Gaining

You might find that some foods make you feel better when dieting, while others should be saved for a time when desired caloric intake is higher. Typically, the foods that constitute someone's diet in a steep caloric deficit will vary greatly from foods that make up the diet of someone who is trying to gain weight. It is not that specific foods push us in one way or the other, but rather that the overall pattern of our diet will reflect our own specific goals at any given time. Let's take a closer look.

As we have discussed, it is much more difficult to get adequate nutrients in a caloric deficit because you are simply consuming fewer calories. For this reason, it is crucial to consume a high quantity of nutrient-dense foods. There is less room for "fun" foods in a caloric deficit. Nutrient-dense foods provide an additional benefit when dieting: they keep you full. Whole foods are often high in volume and fiber, so they help keep you satiated during a time when it seems like your body is always telling you that you are hungry. On the other hand, it can be more of a challenge to eat an excess of these foods when you are in a caloric surplus.

While you might find that you feel best eating a giant salad for at least one meal every day when dieting, it can be difficult just to get down a large volume of food in one sitting if you are trying to gain weight. A good protocol is to slowly increase your intake of higher-calorie foods that might be less nutrient dense when your goal is to gain weight. This will allow you to reach your nutrition goals comfortably, that is, without feeling like you cannot finish your meals.

Just remember that it is not the case that certain foods will help you reach your goals faster but rather that certain foods can be more conducive to comfort and health depending on the stage of your dietary journey. This is just one example of the way that different situations and goals can alter which types of foods should constitute the bulk of your diet.

## The Pursuit of Satisfaction

Satiation describes the biological processes that bring an eating episode to an end. Satiation comes when food in the stomach expands the stomach walls. As food fills the stomach, signals are sent to the brain that indicate that eating should end. Bariatric surgery that shrinks the stomach makes it easier to reach satiation as less food volume is required to expand the stomach and send signals to the brain. On the other hand, satiety describes a state that strongly suggests we restrict from eating until our next meal. Satiety is influenced by factors like fiber, protein, and caloric density of foods. Fats can also help us feel full, but keep in mind that fat is more calorically dense than carbohydrates and protein, so we need to eat more calories when we consume fat to achieve fullness.

Two meals with similar macronutrient compositions can vary hugely in the degree of satiation that they cause. I recently purchased a small prepackaged meal with 9 g fat, 28 g carbs, 21 g protein to satisfy hunger between breakfast and lunch. This macronutrient composition is similar if not the same as the macronutrient composition of many popular protein bars. The meal consisted of lean bison, chicken, rice, and vegetables, filled a 7 in. × 4 in. × 2 in. container and weighed 259 g. Typical protein bars measure 5 in. × 1.5 in. × 0.5 in. and weigh about 60 g. The prepackaged meal, much higher in volume, filled my stomach and made me feel full. The fibrous vegetables and high protein content kept me satiated until my next meal.

Some protein bars are very high in fiber; even though a protein bar does not expand your stomach to tell your brain that the meal is over, the fiber and protein will keep you feeling satiated long after you are done eating.

While the caloric density of both options is probably not enough to keep you satiated for more than a few hours, the impact of volume, fiber, and protein can help you feel full when calories are restricted. Taking advantage of this knowledge also helps when trying to gain weight; you might want to reduce your intake of extremely high-volume, high-fiber foods if you are trying to gain weight.

How exactly is it that fiber, protein, and volume can make us feel full even when calories are low? High-fiber foods are often high in volume, but even when they are not, as in the case of a protein bar, the fiber keeps you full for a long time because it takes longer for the food to be digested and absorbed.

Proteins are complex molecules, and it takes a long time to break them down into their amino acid components. Many people like protein powder supplements for its quick absorption. On the other hand, many of us want the benefit of staying full for a longer amount of time. Although drinking protein shakes when dieting can be a great idea because of their high volume, a protein shake will not keep you satiated for as long as a typical meal, as gastric emptying, digestion, and absorption of liquid meals is faster than solid meals.

Consumption of high-protein meals is filling and effective. If your goal is simply to lose weight, a high-protein diet may be easiest to follow because it is so satiating. When dieting, satiety decreases as leptin is decreased, and hunger increases as ghrelin is increased.

On the other hand, fat is filling because it is calorie dense. Remember that fat has nine calories per gram whereas carbohydrates and protein each have four calories per gram.

Air content (think of popcorn or rice cakes) and water content (think of cucumbers or lettuce) of foods can increase the volume of our meals and consequently increase satiation. As the stomach fills up with food, nerve-stretch receptors send signals to the brain that the meal is over. Ghrelin decreases and leptin increases (more after a carbohydrate-heavy meal than a fat-heavy meal). Cholecystokinin (CCK) and peptide YY (PYY) are produced in the small bowel and released in response to food in the gut to signal fullness.

Foods that have little volume, fiber, or protein will not leave you feeling full after your meal, but if the calorie content of the meal is also low, you are still in good shape if you eat other foods that make you feel full. This is the difference between eating one cookie or chip or piece of candy as opposed to several. A small portion of food that does not contribute to satiation or satiety may be fine, but spending too many of your calories on these foods can leave you feeling much hungrier than you need to be.

Sometimes the hard part is listening to these signals and acting appropriately. Many of us keep eating after we feel full or start eating our next meal when we are not actually hungry. Others may ignore hunger signals and avoid eating even when we are hungry. Flexible dieting takes away the necessity of acting on these signals appropriately. For many of us, it is easier to stick to a set of numbers than to try and guess what our bodies are telling us these numbers should be.

It is normal to feel hungry when you are dieting. Appetite hormones respond to dieting to make us hungry and want to eat more; however, understanding which foods are more satiating can help you suffer less when dieting (and not feel stuffed when trying to gain weight).


## A Balancing Act

There are many small steps that you can take to optimize progress. Each one might have a seemingly negligible impact, but when you do them all together, there will be noticeable difference. For example, if your goal is to retain or gain lean mass, you can increase muscle protein synthesis by consuming protein after workouts, choosing protein sources that are high in leucine, or taking supplements like creatine around workout times. Research is often lacking on topics where the goal is not treating diseases but rather optimizing body composition or performance beyond a normal healthy range. You might find that certain approaches work for you even though research is sparse or has shown an alternate outcome.

On the other hand, you should ask yourself how far you are willing to go in pursuit of your goals. Not only does this require dedication that sometimes borders on obsession, but in some cases, the implementation of so many practices can backfire and impede the progress you want to achieve by adding too much negative stress. As with anything in life, you must love the journey as much as the goal. Many of us want to accomplish dreams yet do not want to put in the work it takes to achieve those dreams.

Successful flexible dieting requires a balancing act. Always keep what means the most to you at the forefront of your focus.

# Eating for Mental Health

You might love eating fish, sweet potato, and vegetables because you love the way it gives you energy for your workouts without making you feel overly full. You might love eating homemade brownies from your mom because it reminds you of happy childhood memories. Both are examples of eating for mental health.

None of my graduate-level nutrition classes ever mentioned eating for mental health. I assume this is because over one-third of American adults are obese, over two-thirds of American adults are overweight or obese, and about one-third of American children and adolescents aged 6 to 19 are overweight or obese. So why encourage consumption of less-nutritious foods that are already consumed excessively by a large portion of individuals?

It is estimated that twenty million women and ten million men suffer from an eating disorder during their lives. It makes sense that nutrition education should focus on nutrient-dense foods when so many of us struggle with excess weight. However, I see two potential areas of improvement here: the first is that mental health is much more difficult to measure than weight. Many of those with eating disorders will live their entire lives undiagnosed. The second is that people who care about nutrition might be more susceptible to obsessing about what they eat and adopt negative eating habits. Despite a lack of research in these areas, common sense suggests that someone who tracks intake is more likely to take it too far than someone who is not tracking his or her intake at all.

Please consider not only your physical health but also your mental health when deciding what to eat.

# 8
# EATING OUT

Many health professionals, fitness gurus, and general gym-goers make it seem like the secret to successful dieting is being prepared. But what happens when you go on vacation or go out to celebrate a special occasion? What happens when your friend gives you a cookie from an expensive bakery or your mom makes you lasagna for dinner? What is the right move? Can you still stay on track if you accept their offers?

Even for the most experienced flexible dieters, there are some foods that are just plain difficult to track. For these foods, the best approach is to estimate as best you can. Even if you are way off, you will likely be closer to reaching your macronutrient intake goals than if you were to totally ignore your diet goals.

You do not have to abandon your diet on special occasions. The worst-case scenario is that there is no nutritional information provided, that you have no food scale, and that you have no idea beforehand what food options you will have. The good news is that you can still stick to your diet by estimating.

## Portions

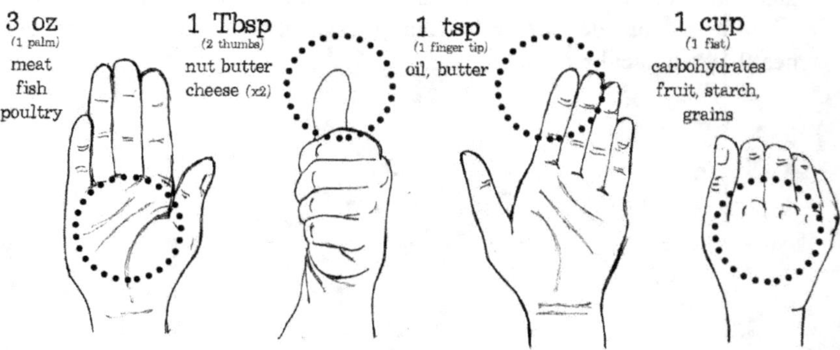


The easiest way is often to look up a database entry for a similar food. Type "homemade chocolate chip cookie" or "homemade beef lasagna" in your food-tracking app or add "nutrition" to the end of either and Google it, and then determine the variant that seems to best fit your intake. Estimate the portion size as best as you can based on experience and the information available from the entries. Once you weigh your food for a while, it becomes easier to estimate portion sizes. When you weigh 4 oz of chicken three hundred times, it becomes much easier to estimate a portion of 4 oz of chicken. For newbies, you might want to refer to a visual chart when estimating portion sizes; such helpful charts can be easily found by performing a quick Google search.

Using visual cues can be an effective shortcut to a diet that benefits both long-term health and short-term fitness goals. To achieve your goals, you do not need to be a slave to meal prep, but you do need to have a good understanding of the nutritional content of food so that you can appropriately estimate calorie and nutrient content on the go. Poor estimation skills can be dangerous. A "handful" of nuts, a "spoonful" of peanut butter, or a "medium" potato can mean very different size portions to different people. Make sure you practice estimating until you become confident in your skills. Practice weighing food for weeks, months, or even years before just winging it.

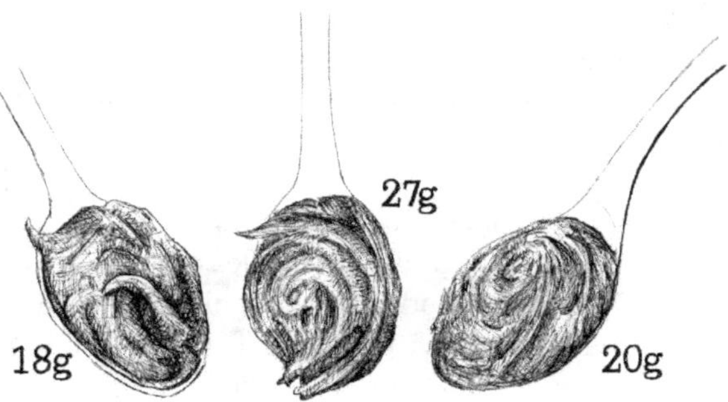


To play it safe, we should overestimate our portions when dieting. Research suggests that we tend to underestimate the size of large, restaurant-type meal portions. Of course, your tendencies might an exception to this, so it is important to consider your own history. Do you have a history of significantly restricting calories? You might need to decrease your estimations from those to which you are accustomed. Have you always struggled to lose weight? You might need to increase your estimations to account for your tendencies.

## Ingredients

Another approach to tracking your dietary intake is to break down the food into its ingredients. This is difficult if you do not know the ingredients. "Chicken sandwich" describes a meal that can have a widely variable macronutrient composition depending on the ingredients. A bun with grilled chicken, tomato, and lettuce is much different from bread stuffed with that same grilled chicken, tomato, lettuce, cheese, avocado, bacon, and mayonnaise. If you order a chicken sandwich, it would be much easier to track the individual ingredients than the meal itself. When the restaurant nutrition data is easily accessible, you can resort to that instead. While the published nutrition data is often inaccurate, it does provide us with a means from which we can estimate.

## Smart Choices

Restaurants that allow you to choose individual ingredients for your meal are key for flexible dieting if you do not want to ask the waiter to make substitutions. If you do not want the fat from sour cream or cheese or the carbohydrates from rice, simply avoid ordering those options. Burritos, bowls, deli sandwiches, and salads are common meal types that you can order this way.

At most restaurants, we have less control over our orders; other times, we lack control over which foods are accessible to us or what is served on our plates. However, we always have at least some degree of control over what we eat. Dieting and working toward physique goals are privileges. If you are ever confronted with food that just does not fit into your diet no matter how much you want it to, remember that you can control what goes into your mouth.

When you are on vacation or at a restaurant, you can stick to your daily macronutrient intake goals by making mindful choices. A "mindful choice" means a choice for which you can estimate the macronutrient and caloric composition. And do not be afraid to ask about preparation techniques or serving sizes. Restaurant meals are often very high in calories and fat. Be on the lookout for excess fat and sugar that often come in the form of toppings, sauces, and dressings.

Keep in mind that a mindful choice is not always a "fun choice." Just because you take a break from diligently tracking your macronutrient intake does not mean you can eat whatever you want. Steer clear of overdoing foods that are low in nutrients to get the most out of your diet. Overall health should take precedence over any short-term diet goals.

When all else fails, you can keep progress moving forward by estimating calories instead of macronutrients. While we cannot always control the ingredients of the meals we are served, we can control the portions we choose to eat. For example, many restaurant menus are full of high-fat choices. In these cases, it can be helpful to choose a low-carb meal so that your meal is not packed with both carbohydrates and fat. Calories are more critical than macronutrient composition for reaching our diet goals, although optimizing macronutrient intake will give you better results than calorie counting alone. If you cannot control the macronutrient composition of the meal, you can still control the calorie content. Do not be afraid to leave some food on your plate.

## What About Alcohol ?

Alcohol provides us with calories but not nutrients. The 2015–2020 US Dietary Guidelines recommend that adults of legal drinking age who consume alcohol regularly should not drink more than one drink per day for women and two drinks per day for men. As defined by the US Dietary Guidelines, one drink consists of 12 fl oz of beer at 5% alcohol, 5 fl oz of wine at 12% alcohol, and 1.5 fl oz of 80 proof distilled spirits at 40% alcohol.

The curve of the association between alcohol consumption and mortality is J-shaped, making it seem like moderate amounts of alcohol (limited as recommended above) are more beneficial than not drinking at all or heavy drinking (which is associated with many negative outcomes, like increased risk of many cancers). However, these findings may be biased by the "sick-quitter" effect. Categorizing individuals who developed illness because of their alcohol intake or who were otherwise negatively affected by alcohol and quit as "non-drinkers" can severely bias study findings to make it look like non-drinkers have poorer health than moderate drinkers, simply because they never developed a serious problem because of their drinking and had to quit. Moreover, the data come from observational studies. People drinking one to two drinks per day might be doing something else to benefit their health. Maybe they are less stressed, for example. A cause-and-effect relationship has not been established.

When we track macronutrients, we use Atwater factors (i.e.

carbohydrates have four calories per gram, protein has four calories per gram, and fat has nine calories per gram). Alcohol has seven calories per gram. Since seven calories per gram is between four calories per gram (as carbohydrates have) and nine calories per gram (as fat has), an easy way to track alcohol is to count 50% of the calories as coming from carbohydrates and 50% as coming from fat. Alternately, you could decide to track it as carbohydrates only or fat only.

For example, a 120-calorie drink can be split into 60/4 = 15 g of carbohydrates and 60/9 = 6.7 g of fat. Alternately, you could count it as 120/4 = 30 g of carbohydrates or 120/9 = 13.3 g of fat.

# 9

# A TIME AND PLACE FOR ALL FOODS

Too many of us fail to reach our fitness and health goals because of an all-or-nothing mentality. Either you eat healthy or you don't. If your meals do not consist of salmon, kale, and quinoa, then you're not trying to be healthy. This mindset is perpetuated not only by a bombardment of marketing from the food industry and in the general media but even by tools that are meant to inform us. Whole and minimally processed foods fill the USDA food pyramid and MyPlate (the current nutrition guide published by the USDA Center for Nutrition Policy and Promotion). As we have mentioned, many of the most popular foods in the US, like french fries, pizza, and snacks like chips and cookies, are absent from these representations of a healthy diet. Are we all failing at being healthy humans if we consume these foods? No, of course not.

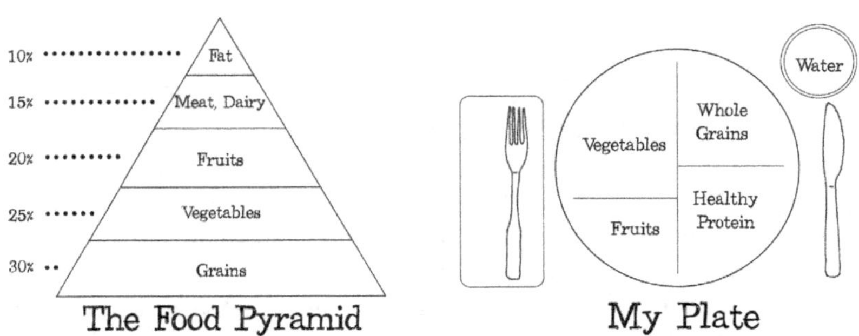


The Food Pyramid          My Plate

Michael Pollan gets it right: "Eat food. Not too much. Mostly plants." But if we don't follow his advice, are our food choices automatically wrong? Many of us love to think in black-and-white terms, but there are so many shades of gray to a healthy diet. Feeling anxious because you feel like you didn't eat enough vegetables today is not what a healthy diet is about. Today in the US, a healthy diet is one that leaves room for some treats and less nutrient-dense foods here and there. A healthy diet is one that leaves room for enjoying your favorite foods.

Most of us do not always eat meals that resemble the USDA MyPlate template, and if we do, we might just be missing out. The plate is a great tool to indicate that most of our diet should come from plant-based foods. Unfortunately, because of the abundance of "junk food" that is constantly shoved in our faces, we do need tools like this to remind us what a balanced diet looks like. However, including foods not depicted on the plate or in the pyramid does not necessarily mean that we have a bad diet and are at an increased risk for disease. Consuming a variety of foods that are easily accessible to us just means that we are human. We are living in a time where much of the food that is accessible to us does not resemble anything on the USDA MyPlate.

Obviously, we do not need to eat junk food, but the reality is that there is so much of it available to us that it is difficult to avoid. For many, avoiding all foods that are processed or prepared by someone else means living in isolation, inevitably turning down offers to enjoy meals with others, and rejecting foods that are provided to us at work, school, and social events.

Additionally, many processed foods are enriched with nutrients and contain preservatives, so not only do they supply us with vitamins and minerals, but they also last longer so we do not need to waste as much. It makes sense for many of us who are on a budget to opt for these foods when grocery shopping. When we adopt an all-or-nothing mentality, we forget that a diet rich in whole foods is not synonymous with a diet consisting of only whole foods. You can eat both fruit and gummy bears, both oats and bread, and still have a nutritious diet. Your body does not set off an alarm when you eat processed foods that tells it to stop functioning properly. A healthy functioning body sees only food and digests and absorbs that food appropriately no matter its ingredients.

While some foods are certainly more nutritious and arguably "better" options to spend your macro budget on, there are additional, personal reasons that can make certain foods better than others, ranging from health diagnoses to personal beliefs. Each reason can be integrated into a flexible dieting approach to make it work for you. Remember that flexible dieting is all about making your diet work with your life—not making your life work with your diet.

If you do not have a personal reason to entirely avoid a specific food, there is no reason to exclude any single food or nutrient from your diet. Yet many of us are afraid of specific foods and think that eliminating them completely from our diets will make us healthier individuals. Let's examine several common culprits.

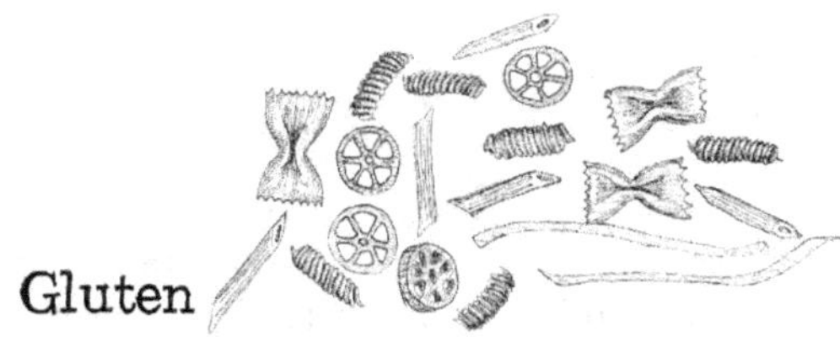

# Gluten

Gluten accounts for most protein in wheat. Foods containing gluten are excellent sources of protein, iron, fiber, and other nutrients, and they are often low in fat. For anyone with a largely plant-based diet, consuming foods high in gluten is a great way to increase protein intake.

If you have celiac disease, gluten sensitivity, or a wheat allergy, you should stay away from gluten. There is also evidence suggesting that individuals with digestive disorders like IBS can relieve symptoms by reducing or eliminating gluten intake. If you do not have any of these diagnoses, gluten is a great source of nutrients that should not be avoided. Consumption of gluten-containing whole grains is associated with reduced risk of conditions such as heart disease, type 2 diabetes, obesity, and some forms of cancer.

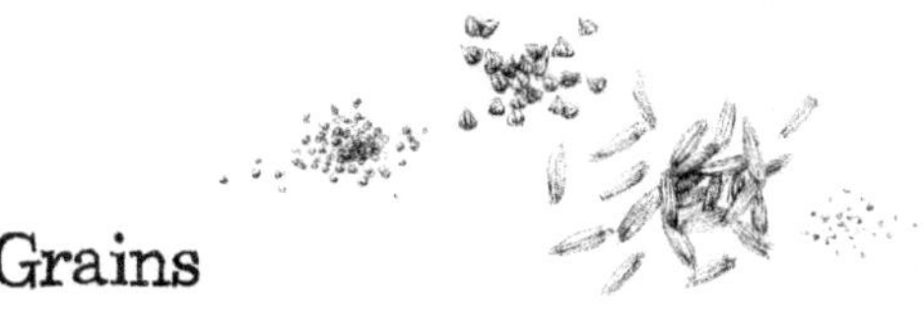

# Grains

Grains are sometimes targeted for more than just their gluten content. The USDA recommends that a balanced diet should be rich in fruit, vegetables, whole grains, and legumes. So where then do grains get a bad reputation? Phytic acid, a substance found in grains, legumes, nuts, and seeds, can bind to certain minerals like iron, zinc, and calcium and prevent their intestinal uptake and decrease their absorption. However, there is no reason to worry about phytic acid if you are consuming whole grains in moderation and eating plenty of other nutrient-dense foods. If phytic-acid-rich foods are a huge staple in your diet, then soaking, sprouting, or fermenting grains can be an effective way to reduce phytic-acid content. While grains can cause digestive distress in some individuals, they are perfectly safe for many of us.

# Bread 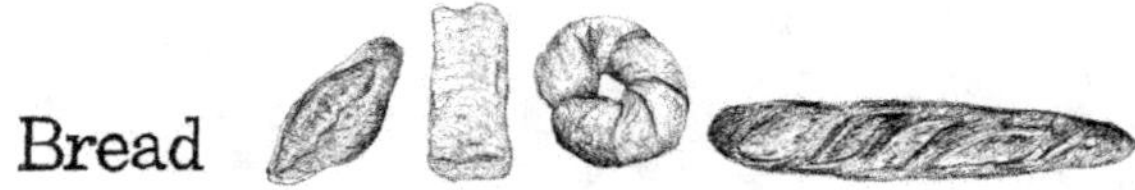

Whole grains will typically give you more fiber, iron, and B vitamins as compared with enriched refined grains. Bread has a faster rate of gastric uptake and absorption than whole grains and is less filling than many whole grains, but it has no inherent negative effect on fat loss or overall health.

Many bread products are labeled as "whole grain" or "multigrain," which is confusing. Often these products are not much less refined than white bread. Whole grains are intact, retaining the endosperm, germ, and bran, but there is no requirement or guideline for what constitutes a "whole-grain food." Wheat bread is typically made with flour and therefore does not contain intact grains, but specialty bread products may contain intact grains. In general, a greater proportion of intact grains translates to greater satiety and a lower glycemic index. Despite what the packaging says, remember to check the nutrition label to see how much fiber and nutrients your bread really contains.

Even though bread is not as satiating as some other sources of carbohydrates, it does not stall fat loss, so simply replacing bread with a lower-glycemic index source will not increase fat loss.

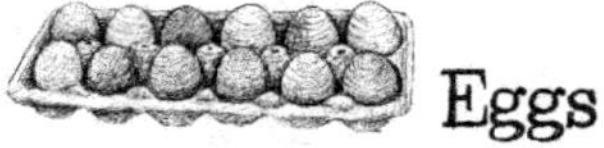 # Eggs

Eggs have a historically controversial reputation due to their cholesterol content. In the past, the American Heart Association has recommended a daily limit of 300 mg of dietary cholesterol. At 185 mg per egg, two eggs put you over this limit. However, this recommendation has been lifted, as high dietary cholesterol does not necessarily equate to high serum cholesterol levels.

The albumen (egg white) is made up of mostly protein and water. One of those proteins, called avidin, binds to the B vitamins in the egg whites and prevents their absorption when raw. Heating processes, including pasteurization, destroy most avidin in the egg white, so absorption of B vitamins is not impaired.

Egg yolk is lower in protein than the albumen but high in the amino acid leucine, which can stimulate muscle protein synthesis. Yolks are mostly fatty acids, cholesterol, and fat-soluble nutrients. A typical chicken egg derives nearly half of its fat from oleic acid (a MUFA), with the next highest fat content coming from saturated fat. PUFAs make up the rest of the egg's fat content. The PUFAs are mostly omega-6 fatty acids in eggs coming from grain-fed chickens, but eggs from chickens with special diets can also have more omega-3 PUFAs in their yolks. Egg yolks are also one of the best sources of choline.

Eggs contain eighteen of the twenty amino acids and are extremely nutrient-dense foods. There is no reason to fear eggs or their yolks.

# Dairy 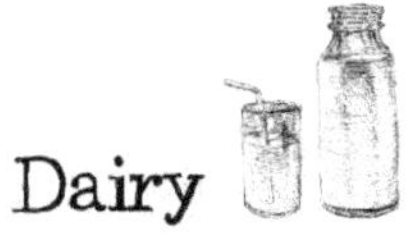

Dairy is high in protein and calcium. There are many myths that suggest that dairy makes us bloat or—worse—that it makes us fat. It is possible that these myths originated because many of us are in fact lactose intolerant. Indeed, if you are lactose intolerant, then consuming dairy will probably cause bloating and discomfort, among other possible symptoms. But that does not mean it will make us gain significant fat (as long as overall calorie intake is not at a surplus). It just means that those of us who are lactose intolerant risk stomach upset and other digestive issues when we consume dairy products.

During the agricultural revolution, agriculture replaced hunting and gathering, and farmers started learning how to make yogurt and cheese, which both have lower lactose levels than milk. These can be good dairy sources of protein and calcium for those of us who do not do well with high levels of lactose.

Low-fat dairy is recommended by the USDA as an essential part of a balanced diet. While full-fat dairy products are high in saturated fat, they also deserve a place in a balanced diet.

Today, dairy products are so widely consumed that it is difficult to avoid them. Unless you have an intolerance or an allergy, you do not have to worry about asking, "Is it dairy-free?" Many dairy products that are already high in calcium are also fortified with vitamin D, which can be difficult to get in adequate amounts from food alone. Like eggs, milk has eighteen of the twenty amino acids.

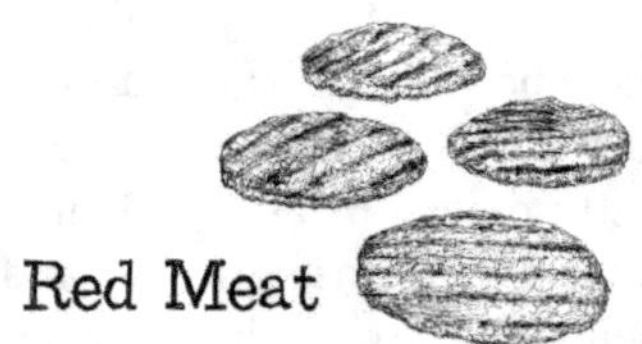

# Red Meat

Red meat contains heme iron, which can increase the formation of carcinogenic N-nitroso-compounds (NOC) in the digestive tract. Several NOCs are potential human carcinogens. However, red meat is also high in several vitamins and minerals, such as B vitamins, iron, zinc, and phosphorus and all amino acids. Beef liver is one of the most nutrient-dense foods we can eat.

A 2016 meta-analysis by O'Connor et al. found that eating a serving of red meat three times per week did not influence blood pressure, cholesterol, or triglyceride levels. People fear the saturated fat, cholesterol, and sodium content in red meat. However, if eaten in moderation, these attributes need not inhibit our dietary choices.

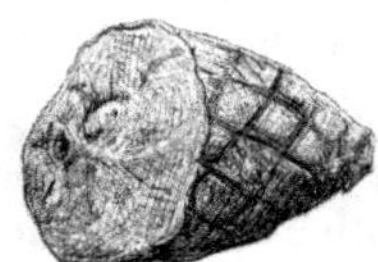

# Processed Meat

Processing meat by adding nitrites or nitrates to cure it or by smoking it to an extent that carcinogenic compounds like N-nitroso-compounds (NOC) and polycyclic aromatic hydrocarbons (PAH) are formed is a different story. Note that the source of nitrate does not matter. Some processed meats advertise themselves as "nitrate-free," but they are preserved with celery juice; celery is rich in nitrates. Grilling or barbecuing or other high-temperature cooking can also produce carcinogens like heterocyclic aromatic amines (HAA) and PAHs. What is the level of risk? Here is an excerpt written by Stacy Simon for cancer.org: "Overall, the lifetime risk of someone developing colon cancer is 5%. To put the numbers into perspective, the increased risk from eating the amount of processed meat in the study would raise average lifetime risk to almost 6%." We are talking about 50 g of processed meat per day to get this level of increased risk.

# Cooked Food 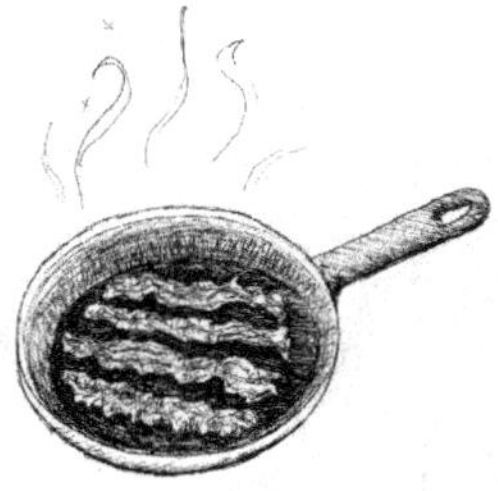

Some raw foodists claim that cooking destroys enzymes in food and that we should only eat raw; however, there is no reason to avoid cooked food. Cooked food has many benefits, like making certain nutrients more available to us and making food taste better and more easily digested. Lutein and beta-carotene content is higher in cooked spinach. Cooking spinach can also decrease the amount of chemicals that inhibit absorption of calcium and iron. Carotenoid and lycopene contents are higher in cooked tomatoes than raw. On the other hand, too much boiling can decrease nutrient content, and blackening or charring is linked to the formation of carcinogens. It is wise to cook using a variety of methods to ensure a balance of nutrients in your diet. When it comes to cooking—just like with anything else—variety is best.

# Sugar 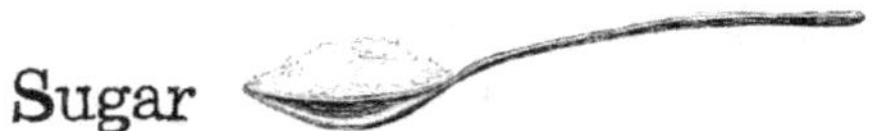

Contrary to popular belief, sugar is not the source of all our problems. First, there is a difference between glucose, which is found in every cell in our bodies, and fructose, which is not produced by the body. Fructose can only be metabolized by the liver. If we consume small amounts of fructose, such as the amounts found in fruit, it will be converted to glycogen and stored in the liver to use for energy later. However, if we consume more fructose than the liver can handle, the extra is stored in adipose tissue (body fat).

There is also a difference between fruit and fruit juice. It would be nearly impossible to overload the liver with fructose by eating fruit. Drinking juice (or soda), on the other hand, is an easy way to consume fructose and other sugar in very large amounts. And when you see high-fructose corn syrup on a nutrition label, it describes a blend of glucose and fructose, the same molecules that sucrose is broken down into before it is absorbed by our intestines.

Typically, some water is removed from fruit juice during processing, so even if the juice says, "no sugar added," you are getting a much more calorie- and sugar-dense beverage than if you were to juice the fruit at home. However, freshly squeezed juice is not as amazing as it is often made out to be. Depending on how the fruit is juiced, the juicing process can virtually eliminate the fiber content. You are better off blending your fruit if you want to drink it so that all the nutrients are retained. But if you are looking for a quick, concentrated dose of sugar, perhaps before or after a long workout or a race, then juice is a great idea.

Fruit supplies us with fiber, vitamins, minerals, antioxidants, and naturally occurring sugars. High fruit intake has been associated with reduced risk of heart disease, heart attack, and stroke. Fruit is also filling. In many cases, fresh fruit is a better choice than dried fruit, not only because sugar is often added onto the dried fruit but also because dried fruit is less filling. Just imagine how many dried apricots it would take to fill your stomach versus fresh ones.

The danger of added sugars is that they can increase calories by large amounts while adding no additional nutrients. Large amounts of any kind of sugar can increase insulin resistance and even increase risk of developing diabetes. There is even evidence that elevated insulin levels are related to cancer.

However, people who obsess about how many grams of sugar they should aim for per day are missing the picture: remember the goal of flexible dieting is to get calories from a variety of sources.

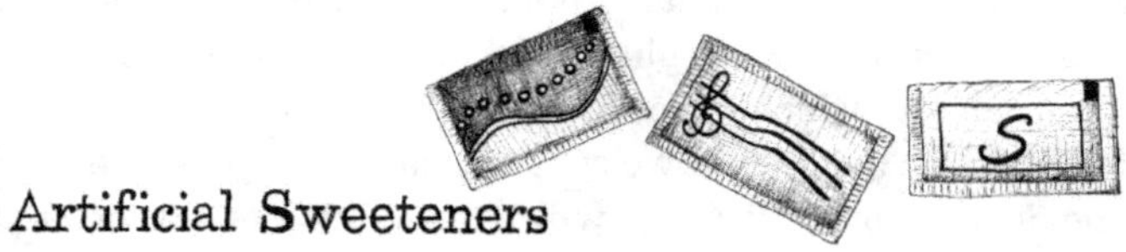

## Artificial Sweeteners

Artificial sweeteners can help reduce sugar and overall caloric intake, but they can also cause digestive issues, interfere with gut bacteria, and cause cravings. The various types of artificial sweeteners can have different risks and benefits and may also affect you differently than other people.

Associations that have been found between artificial sweeteners and negative health outcomes (e.g. daily consumption of diet soda has been linked to an increased risk for metabolic syndrome and type 2 diabetes) might have little to do with the effects of artificial sweeteners themselves. Individuals who tend to consume them may also tend to have other behaviors that ultimately increase their risk of these outcomes. For instance, drinking a diet soda can contribute to a preference and/or cravings for very sweet foods. It might be an overconsumption of sugar or a general caloric surplus that can lead to negative outcomes. If you track your intake and do not let artificial sweeteners influence the rest of your intake, then artificial sweeteners can be a useful tool when dieting. However, if you do not currently use artificial sweeteners, there is no reason to start.

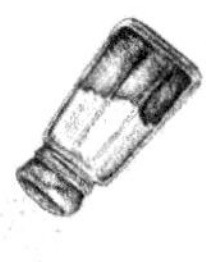

# Salt

We have been led to believe that high sodium intake translates to high blood pressure and increased risk of heart disease. The USDA guidelines recommend less than 2,400 mg of sodium per day for healthy adults and 1,500 mg or less for individuals over the age of fifty or at risk for hypertension. A mere teaspoon of salt provides 2,300 mg of sodium; however, there is a lack of research associated with reducing sodium intake to these low levels.

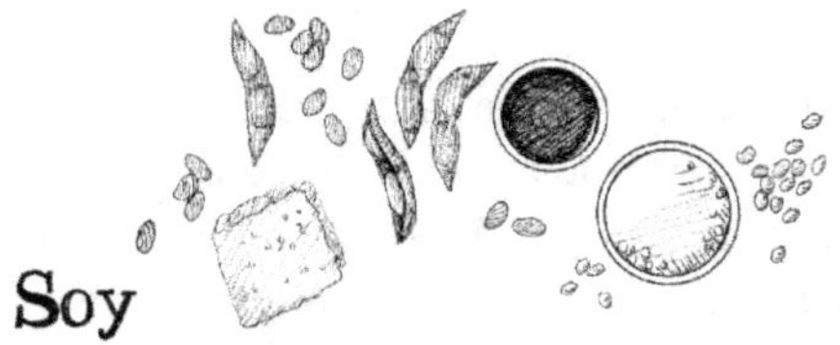

# Soy

Soy, listed as a one of the "foods that fights cancer" by the American Institute of Cancer Research (AICR), contains phytochemicals and active compounds that could lower cholesterol, protect against cancer, affect blood glucose levels, act as antioxidants, and stop cancer cells from spreading or progressing to tumors.

Phytoestrogens like isoflavones have a mild estrogenic effect. By blocking excess production of actual estrogen, isoflavones may stop cancer. The misconception that soy intake can lead to cancer comes from the fact that high levels of estrogens are linked to breast cancer (not phytoestrogens).

Studies that have found negative health outcomes from soy were studying soy supplements, not soy as food. But the amount of soy isolate found in snacks and supplements is safe. The AICR references seven soy bars a day as the upper amount of what is considered safe per day.

Soy-based products are excellent sources of plant-based protein, and if consumed as part of a balanced diet, soy's benefits far outweigh any potential harm.

# 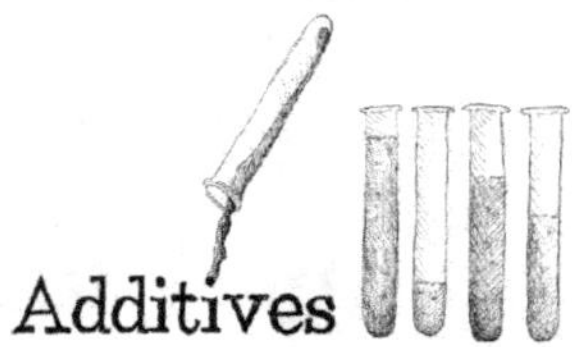Additives

More foods are processed than you might think. Cut, cooked, canned, frozen, or packaged foods are all processed to some extent. Adding sweeteners, oils, spices, preservatives, and coloring requires processing. Prepackaged snack foods, deli meat, and microwaveable meals require some of the highest levels of processing of all.

Several food dyes have been shown to be contaminated with carcinogens or otherwise cause cancer in rats. For instance, a potential carcinogen, 4-methylimidazole (4-MEI), is formed during the manufacture of caramel coloring. At the same time, food coloring is used in very small amounts. Most of us do not drink plain food coloring.

Preservatives in food provide protection against reactive oxygen species (ROS) that are associated with cancer, cardiovascular disease, and aging. They also make food taste better. Ascorbic acid, a common preservative used to prevent ripening and decay, may inhibit the formation of some carcinogens. However, nitrosamines from nitrates, which prevent the growth of harmful bacteria, and butylated hydroxyanisole (BHA) and butylated hydroxytoluene (BHT), which can prevent fats from oxidizing and becoming rancid, are potentially carcinogenic in large amounts.

It is likely that the benefits of preservatives outweigh the potential problems considering that they are not consumed in very large amounts relative to our total food intake.

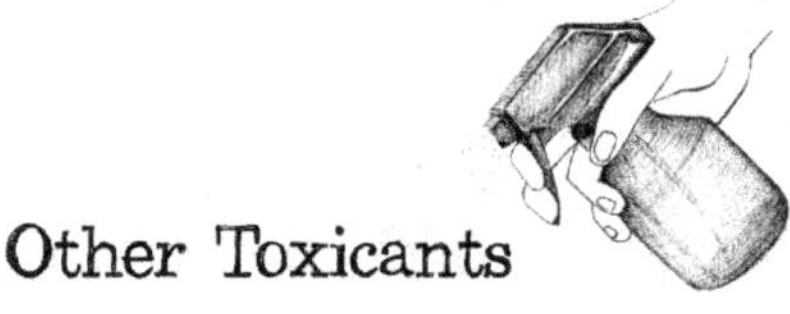

# Other Toxicants

Although it is used to describe any toxic substance, the term "toxin" means a toxic substance that is produced by a living organism. "Toxicant" is a more appropriate term to describe all toxic substances.

Pesticides are often found on produce that we consume as trace residues. While we certainly do not want to eat pure pesticides for lunch, an apple with some trace residues is still an apple. The "dirty dozen" is a list of foods that are supposed to have the most pesticides because they lack a peel that you can remove to "take off" the toxicants. However, there is a lack of research on benefits from swapping out conventional "dirty dozen" produce for organic or on risks from consuming the "dirty dozen." Families who feel that they cannot afford organic produce often turn to other cheap sources of calories, like fast food, packaged snack foods, and soda. Conventional produce would be a much more nutrient-dense option.

Similarly, there are people who eliminate fish from their diet because they are afraid of mercury and other toxicants. Unfortunately, they miss out on an excellent source of omega-3 fatty acids and other nutrients.

Toxicants can be found in or on virtually any food. Nitrates, solanins, mushroom poisons, raw soybeans and rapeseeds, fava beans, and raw cabbage-family vegetables are all potentially toxic. Cyanogenic glycosides in sweet potatoes and stone fruit can cause gastrointestinal inflammation. Glucosinolates in onions, cabbage, peanuts, and soybeans can cause goiter, impaired metabolism, and decreased iodine and protein uptake. Phenols in most fruits and vegetables, tea, coffee, cereals, soybeans, and potatoes can diminish thiamine and raise cholesterol. Oxalates in spinach and tomatoes can reduce the solubility of iron, zinc, and calcium. Glycoalkaloids in potatoes and tomatoes can negatively affect the central nervous system; cause kidney inflammation, cancer, birth defects; and decrease iron uptake. Lectins in cereals, soybeans, and potatoes can cause intestinal inflammation and reduce nutrient uptake/absorption. Coumarins in celery, parsley, parsnips, and figs are light-activated carcinogens and can cause skin irritation. The list goes on.

These are all natural foods, modified in no way, and organic versions can have the same effects as conventional. I could write a separate book about all the possible toxicants in foods that we like to call "healthy.". The key to remember is that toxicity is a function of dose.

## The Dose Makes the Poison 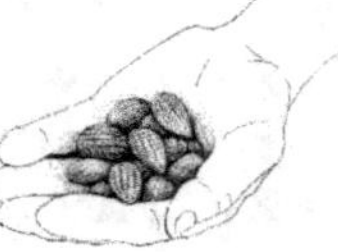

Plastics, fabrics, buildings, and even the air we breathe can expose us to dangerous chemicals. Polybrominated diphenyl ethers (PBDEs) are used in plastics, textiles, building materials, cars, and more. PBDEs have hormone-disrupting effects on estrogen and thyroid hormone. Polychlorinated biphenyl (PCB) was banned in the 1970s but is stable and remains in our environment. PCBs generate dioxins when burned. Phthalates are chemicals added to plastic to increase its durability, flexibility, and longevity. They are also endocrine disruptors, meaning that they interfere with hormones. Unfortunately, the list of chemicals that we are exposed to that can cause negative health effects is exhaustive.

I do not mention these things to scare you but to illustrate that food is not as scary as it may seem. Eliminating entire foods or groups of foods from our diets is the dietary equivalent of living in a bubble to escape all the chemicals to which we are exposed.

Unless you have a health issue that prevents you from eating certain foods, there is no need to eliminate any food—just as there is no need to eliminate buildings or outside air from your life. All foods should be consumed in moderation as part of a balanced diet. Very few of us have a farm where we get 100% of our food. The rest of us need to consume food that was grown or handled by someone else. While specific foods may be avoided for personal reasons, there is no reason for all of us to eliminate any one food from our diets. Our time would be better spent focusing on which foods to fill our diet with rather than obsessing over eliminating or limiting our intake of certain foods.

While the negative effects of any one food are typically negligible, they can add up. It is essential to make sure that the bulk of your diet comes from nutrient-dense, whole foods. For example, if your diet is full of plant-based foods sprinkled with bacon and some diet soda, you are in good shape. But if your diet is full of bacon and diet soda with the occasional fruit or vegetable sprinkled in, it is a good idea to regroup and think about making some changes.

Excessive intake of nutrient-poor, highly palatable foods usually leads to at least one of two things: excessive weight gain, if overall intake is excessive, or lack of adequate nutrients, if nutrient-dense foods are not consumed in addition to the low-nutrient foods. Either case may result in poor health outcomes. We know that overeating in general is associated with weight gain, but overeating nutrient-poor foods despite undereating overall is also not optimal. Growing up, it was not unusual for me to eat ice cream, chocolate, and prepackaged brownies or cookies all in the same day, yet I was always underweight. I was missing out on adequate nutrients. Why no doctor or coach thought to mention diet as a cause of my fainting episodes, general fatigue, and lack of interest in physical activity is beyond me.

While it is much easier to eat too many french fries than to eat too many bananas, any food consumed excessively can give you problems, whether it be digestive issues or major health diagnoses. Even water, which makes up roughly half of our body weight, can be lethal if we drink it to extreme excess. Flexible dieting fights against excess not with restriction but with variety.

When we eliminate foods from or add foods to our diet because of studies that aim to correlate the consumption of specific foods with obesity or disease, we are missing the boat completely. The entire dietary pattern must be considered. Unfortunately, these are the studies that are funded and the results that become sensationalized headlines. Headlines with direct cause-and-effect relationships garner our attention. We like to read headlines like "garlic prevents cancer," as they are consistent with a quick-fix mentality, rather than headlines like "balance is healthy."

## A Time and A Place

I do not have children, but if I am lucky enough to have a child one day, I do not think I will feel comfortable buying him or her very highly palatable, high-fat, high-sugar, high-sodium foods and beverages, like pastries, candy, chocolate, pizza, french fries, chips, and soft drinks. However, I will not object if my child wanted any of these things on a special occasion. After all, birthday cake is meant for birthdays! There is a balance between living in fear of certain foods and feeling guilty after eating them versus incorporating these foods excessively into our diets. Flexible dieting is all about finding that balance.

The bliss point is the amount of an ingredient (usually salt, sugar, or fat) that optimizes the palatability of a food. The human brain reacts to delicious food by releasing the neurotransmitter dopamine. Dopamine can be released after a huge variety of "rewarding" tasks, such as exercising, accomplishing a goal, getting likes on social media, meditating, doing certain types of drugs, achieving "group flow," gambling, playing video games, doing action sports, and attending concerts. Perhaps dopamine is our one true motivator in life.

Salt, sugar, and fat used to be rarities in our diet. Now companies take advantage of our internal reward system to maximize their profits. Everything from chips to video games is designed to create this reward response, to create an "addiction." If we can incorporate these foods into our diet as they were meant to be and not as the main staples of our diet, then we are on track. If you have trouble adhering to an appropriate "dose" of certain foods, then you might find that eliminating them is helpful if not necessary for you to achieve a healthy balance.

Indeed, we need to keep special what is meant to be special. Enjoying dessert with friends or family is special. Eating a pint of ice cream paired with an entire package of cookies alone is not special; it is excessive. Avoiding dessert for your entire life does not make you superior to everyone else who "gives in" to these temptations; it just means you have an unnecessarily restrictive diet. There is a balance that exists for each of us. Remember our budget. If we continually purchase luxury items, we end up in debt. If we never purchase luxury items, we inevitably miss out on social or personal pleasures. Find that what makes sense for your budget, and stick to it.

There is more to a balanced diet than simply avoiding excess. When we eliminate entire food groups, we miss out on some of what nature has to offer us, and we risk consuming too little of certain foods and too much of others. Unless you have a negative physical or mental reaction to a food, there is no reason to remove it from your life. There is indeed a time and place in your life for all foods that you enjoy.

# 10
# MEAL TIMING

Of the many claims about meal timing, one of the most popular is that we should avoid or limit consumption of carbohydrates—or anything at all—at night. This claim assumes that food is somehow more fattening at night. Contrary to what such claims suggest, your body does not say, "Hey, it's 8:00 pm! Let's change the value of a calorie!" While there are additional factors to consider, like insulin sensitivity and circadian rhythms, body composition and weight are largely unaffected by when or how often we eat. However, when and how often we eat can affect factors like performance and satiety, which can in turn affect dietary adherence. Because adherence to your diet is ultimately the key predictor of success, meal timing can help determine the outcome of your diet.

Although total daily intake is the most significant dietary factor in the quest to lose fat or gain muscle, there is still some truth to nutrient timing leaving an impact on our physique and health goals.

## Pre-Workout Nutrition

To maximize muscle protein synthesis and energy levels and to minimize muscle tissue breakdown, it is important to pay attention to nutrient timing around workouts on days that you train. Your ideal pre-workout meal will depend on the type and duration of exercise, but carbohydrates should typically be the focus before workouts. Some people also like to eat or drink something intra-workout, like some simple sugars for added energy. This is typically not necessary unless your workouts are very long, intense, or both. After a workout, dietary protein should be prioritized to stimulate muscle protein synthesis.

A balanced meal with some of each of the three macronutrients and plenty of micronutrients eaten before a workout can provide sufficient fuel. Depending on the activity, a snack of quick-digesting carbohydrates, like a rice cake, honey, or fruit, can give a boost if consumed about thirty minutes beforehand. Some individuals prefer to work out in a fasted state, such as in the morning before eating anything for breakfast. These individuals might want to consider eating a bigger meal before bed or grabbing a quick snack or at least some electrolytes and water before their workout. Personal preference should be the deciding factor for when to plan your resistance training or cardio sessions in relation to your food consumption.

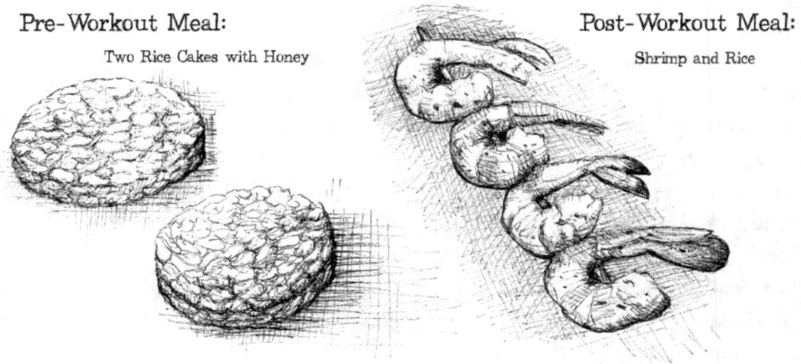



Many people will find that they do not need to interrupt their workouts to eat or drink calories for fuel, while people who train for hours will certainly benefit from ingesting calories during their workouts. Especially for athletes who are competing in races or competitions, electrolytes, glucose, water, and even fat can be extremely helpful for supplying the body with adequate fuel. For the rest of us, ingesting calories during a workout is likely unnecessary and may even cause digestive discomfort.

You may have heard about a post-workout "anabolic window" during which we need to refuel our bodies to maximize progress. Protein intake after a workout helps to maximize the synthesis of protein in our bodies. Muscle protein synthesis increases the thickness and number of muscle fibers, leading to muscle growth. However, research suggests that this anabolic window is rather long in untrained individuals (48–72 hours) but also quite long in trained individuals (approximately 8 hours). Nevertheless, many prefer to eat something long before that window is over. Exercise puts us in a catabolic state, meaning complex molecules, like those that make up muscle tissue, are breaking down. Ingesting calories will help us not only get back into a state of repair and building but also help us to feel refueled after a workout. There is no use in waiting hours to eat just because the research says we can, but there is also no use stressing about drinking a protein shake immediately after a workout just because a guru told us we should.

Until recently, 20–25 g of protein was thought to be the ideal amount of protein to stimulate muscle protein synthesis after a workout, but recent research suggests that 40 g protein post-workout may be superior when it comes to stimulating muscle protein synthesis.

Muscle growth occurs when muscle protein synthesis exceeds muscle protein breakdown for a long period of time. Protein alone triggers muscle protein synthesis, but protein plus resistance training is superior. Not only is exercise catabolic, but it is also insulin-sensitizing, so before, during, and after workouts are all good times to consume carbohydrates because they will be quickly used and absorbed. We also oxidize glucose for fuel and store it as glycogen. However, research suggests that overall daily intake is what matters, as opposed to the precise times when we consume the carbohydrates.

In fact, research seems to indicate that many of the benefits we get from following nutrient timing around workouts are short term. Long-term benefits come from total calorie and macronutrient intake per day, not per meal. If you forget to eat after a workout but have a nice balanced meal before the day is over, then your body will end up getting the proper nutrition needed for recovery. You might need to pay extra attention to pre-workout and post-workout meal timing if you are dieting, simply because it isn't fun to work out hungry or tired. There's no reason to make dieting more uncomfortable than it needs to be by fasting before or after workouts and feeling unnecessarily drained as a result.

When it comes to pre-workout nutrition, the most important potential benefit is psychological. Some people might give different levels of effort with or without 100 g of carbs before their workout. It all comes down to what helps you personally. If you feel good and can finish your workouts and make the progress you want to make, there is no reason to stress about pre- and post-workout meal timing.

## Macronutrient Timing

Macronutrient timing is not as complicated as we make it out to be. Balanced meals provide benefits from all three macronutrients, but for healthy individuals, there are very few risks and benefits associated with consuming specific macronutrients at specific times.

There is a myth that our bodies can only absorb a set amount of protein at one time. The body is amazing at adapting to stress, so this is not an issue with which we need to be particularly concerned. Research has shown that dividing protein intake into fewer or more meals is not associated with differences in protein retention. There is no definitive, maximum amount of protein that we can absorb at one time and above which any additional protein is "wasted." Ideally, you should aim for some protein as part of each meal to help with satiety and muscle protein synthesis, but you will manage just fine no matter how many meals you eat per day or when you consume your protein.

Old school bodybuilding and popular diet philosophy tell us that carbohydrates should be consumed in the morning and that fat should be consumed at night. The idea is that we are more insulin sensitive upon waking and can "better metabolize" carbohydrates, while fat takes longer to digest and will keep us full overnight. However, eating carbohydrates at night will not cause any issues in individuals who do not have diabetes or other major diagnoses, and eating fat at night will not necessarily keep you full. Moreover, individuals with diabetes should be more concerned with consistent consumption of carbohydrates to keep blood sugar levels at an appropriate level. Carbohydrates can certainly be consumed at night in moderation even for those with diabetes. A normal portion of low-glycemic carbohydrates with some protein and fat at night is different than gobbling pancakes covered in syrup.

The glycemic index (GI) of a food is a number that indicates how the food will affect blood glucose levels. While general GIs are assigned to specific foods, a food's effect on blood glucose levels depends on a variety of factors, including ripeness, method of cooking, temperature, storage, processing, and individual insulin resistance. For example, cooled and reheated potatoes may have a lower glycemic index than freshly cooked potatoes. Different varieties of potatoes may have different glycemic indices as well.

There is something beyond the glycemic index that also needs to be considered: the glycemic load (GL). Unlike GI, GL depends on the serving size. To find the GL, multiple the GI by the number of carbohydrates in grams and then divide by 100. The GL of your entire meal can vary hugely depending on what you eat. For example, the GL of a serving of honey or syrup alone will differ from the GL of syrup on pancakes, which will differ from the GL of a serving of honey on chicken.

Countless people have told me that they are (1) avoiding carbohydrates, (2) avoiding high-glycemic carbohydrates, or (3) avoiding carbohydrates at night to either lose weight or be healthier. It turns out that these approaches have little if any effect on weight loss or health in individuals who are already healthy. In general, for those in good health, it is not the timing of food consumed that matters for weight loss but rather the quantity of food consumed.

However, while factors like GI have little effect on body composition, they can affect performance in the gym and everyday life. If your energy levels are low, it might be a matter not of getting enough food but of when you eat. The brain runs on glucose, so forgetting to eat for several hours can result in fatigue from low blood sugar. There is even evidence that blood sugar levels can influence self-control.

## Circadian Clock

Although eating at night versus during the day does not have a dramatic impact on body composition, our bodies do in fact know the difference between night and day. Our circadian biological clock tells us whether it is night or day through rhythms that are approximately 24 hours long. These circadian rhythms are controlled by the suprachiasmatic nucleus (SCN), a part of the brain that responds to light and dark signals. There is evidence of an active circadian clock in several organs with roles involved in nutrition, including the stomach, intestines, pancreas, and liver. The same meal consumed at different times during the day or night can have different effects on the body.

Circadian rhythms can be disrupted due to shift work, jet lag, sleep disorders, and blindness. Short-term effects of disrupted circadian rhythm can include increased blood pressure, decreased blood glucose control, and changes in hunger hormone levels, while long-term disruption of circadian rhythms is associated with weight gain and metabolic diseases like type 2 diabetes.

Especially for those of us who are dieting, meal timing can affect quality of sleep, which can in turn affect diet and health goals. Diets that are high in protein and very low in carbohydrates may lead to restlessness, and severe caloric deficits can lead to extreme hunger, which can in turn lead to insomnia. In these cases, consuming a balanced meal before bed may improve sleep quality. As insulin release promotes the conversion of tryptophan to serotonin, a high-carbohydrate meal before bed may make it easier to sleep than a low-carbohydrate meal.

Lack of sleep in general is associated with increased levels of cortisol and visceral adipose tissue, decreased performance in daily activities, and impaired glucose control. Keep in mind that we are talking about correlations, not cause-and-effect relationships. Decreased sleep can lead to weight gain, primarily through decreased expenditure and increased intake. The best rule for sleep is to get enough so that you feel well rested. A common guidelines is to aim for 7–8 hours per night, but the exact number of hours required for this may vary from individual to individual.

Despite evidence that we are more insulin sensitive in the morning or that hypertrophy signaling might be higher later in the day, reorganizing your diet and exercise schedule based on whatever you think is optimal for your circadian rhythm should not be undertaken if the result has a severely negative impact on the rest of your life. If you have obligations during "peak" times for training or eating, then planning to eat or exercise at this time obviously is not the best fit for you.

## Meals per Day

You may have heard somewhere that a trick to losing weight is to eat small meals throughout the day. Eating small, frequent meals can help prevent you from feeling like you are starving in between meals, but many people simply prefer to continue eating until they are full. Fewer, larger meals might work better for these individuals. On the other hand, if you are someone who overdoes it and ends up eating everything in sight if you go too long in between meals, then small, frequent meals might work best for you. Similarly, smaller, frequent meals can be a great option when you are trying to gain weight so that you can avoid feeling uncomfortably stuffed after a large meal. Nevertheless, some people still prefer to eat fewer, larger meals and to wait until they start to feel hungry before their next meal.

Myths pertaining to nutrient absorption and metabolism state that eating too much at one time is less than ideal because our bodies can only absorb a set amount of nutrients at one time and that eating small, frequent meals will increase your metabolism. As discussed earlier, the body is extremely adaptive, and there is no maximum capacity beyond which nutrients from additional food will be "wasted." Eating frequently does not increase your metabolic rate; eating frequently is simply an effective weight-loss strategy for some if it staves off hunger and decreases overall caloric intake. What matters is that you hit your overall goals regardless of how many meals it takes you to get there.

## Meal Timing Cannot Make You Fat

There are people who will tell you to fill up at breakfast so you do not overeat at night, and there are others who will tell you to eat more calories at night to retain more muscle. The truth is that there is no one-size-fits-all approach. Whatever meal-timing approach helps you stick to your daily calorie and nutrient goals is the "right" approach for you. Meal timing and frequency are extra layers that can either guide your diet toward success or cause unnecessary anxiety. There is no reason to make your diet extra complicated by imposing unnecessary guidelines. On the other hand, if structure throughout the day helps you, whether it involves planning three square meals a day or six smaller meals, then stick to a daily meal schedule.

If you do not typically eat late at night and try it once, then you might notice that you weigh more the next morning than you do when you do not eat late at night. This does not mean that eating late at night makes you gain fat. It just means that there is more food going through your digestive system than usual. In other words, there is more water weight, not more body fat. Try weighing yourself before and after you eat any meal. It should come as no surprise that when you add matter into your body, you weigh more, as weight is defined as a body's relative mass or the quantity of matter that it contains.

Each morning we wake up lighter than we were when we fell asleep because we exhale water vapor and carbon dioxide, we sweat, and we do not eat or drink anything when we sleep. Then we use the bathroom and decrease our weight even more. Throughout the day, our weight increases as we consume food and beverages. Even if we consume an excess of calories such that some of it is stored as fat, we can later use this fat as energy via fat oxidation. To effectively gain body fat, we need to consume excess calories over and over and over. Daily fluctuations should not be confused with significant changes in body fat mass or lean mass.

# 11
# YOUR GOALS

Flexible dieting can help you achieve any health and fitness goal, from losing twenty pounds, to increasing your personal record on bench press by twenty pounds, to feeling more comfortable eating out at restaurants. Of course, the first step to accomplishing your goal is to figure out what that goal is. From there, you can determine the steps it will take to get there with target dates, and finally, you can follow the path that you have carved out for yourself.

A SMART goal is defined as a goal that is specific, measurable, attainable, realistic, and time-based. The idea is to start with a vague goal like "be more confident" or "get healthier" or "lose fat" and then take it one step further to come up with a SMART goal. For example, "lose fat" might become "lose twenty pounds in five months."

Next, write out the steps it will take for you to accomplish your goal. Let's continue with our "lose twenty pounds in five months" example. Note that two individuals with the same goal can have two completely different sets of steps to get there. This is just one example.

## SMART Goal: Lose Twenty Pounds in Five Months

**Steps:**
1. Track dietary intake every day, and aim to end each day within 10 grams of daily fat, carbohydrate, and protein goals.
2. Complete four to five hours of strength training per week.
3. Complete one hour of cardio per week.
4. Aim to lose one pound per week. Decrease intake or increase expenditure each week that one pound was not lost.

Finally, start working on these steps. Each day, choose which steps you need to work on to stay on track toward the bigger goal. At the end of each day, reflect and acknowledge the progress you made. What are you proud of? What can you do better tomorrow? Once a week, regroup and see if you need to make any changes to your game plan.

Now that we have brainstormed a little bit about goal setting, let's see how flexible dieting can help us accomplish some of these goals.

# Performance

Health-related performance goals can be anything from breathing easier to smashing a new personal record in the gym. Whatever your specific goal is, flexible dieting can help to ensure you are getting proper nutrition to support your objectives. Common performance goals include strength, endurance, flexibility, and mobility. Each of these goals requires adequate nutrient intake.

Increasing strength in a caloric surplus is easier than increasing strength at caloric maintenance or in a caloric deficit, but all are possible. More food means more energy, which can mean more strength. In the short term, this might seem straightforward; however, some strength athletes take this approach too far and end up gaining excessive fat, leading to negative health outcomes. In the long term, these negative effects can ultimately backfire and decrease performance. Many strength athletes need high protein and carbohydrate intake unless they want to try a ketogenic diet and use fat for energy. See what works for you and adapt accordingly.

Endurance athletes require much higher amounts of carbohydrates for energy, unless they are using a ketogenic approach. Because endurance athletes burn so many calories overall, they generally need a much higher overall caloric intake as well.

All athletes need to consume a diet that is high in nutrient-dense foods and pay careful attention to micronutrients, especially electrolytes. If your goals are purely performance based, you might not even need to weigh food or track your intake accurately. Estimating and paying attention to nutrient timing could be all that is needed to reach and even surpass your performance goals. Performance athletes should pay careful attention to nutrient intake before, during, and after workouts to optimize performance, recovery, and progress.

To reach any performance goal, flexible dieting should be accompanied by appropriate exercise and training. Regular exercise, even if unrelated to your specific goal, can help to reduce risk of diseases and to strengthen bones and muscle, which in turn will help you increase performance in your sport(s) and everyday life. Finally, proper rest should be prioritized just as high as exercise or diet.

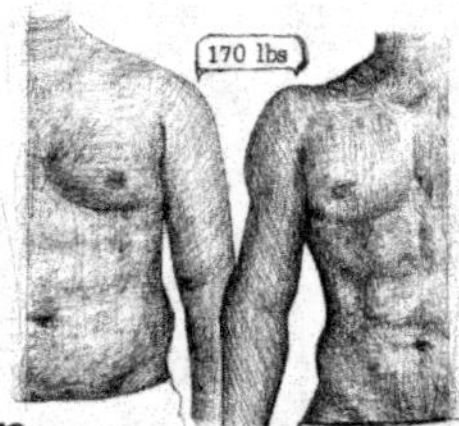


# Body Composition

We mentioned that we can achieve our weight goals through diet only, but can we achieve health and physique goals through diet only? To maximize long-term health, physical activity is necessary. If you want to be the same shape but smaller or larger, you can achieve this through diet alone, although exercise can make it easier by increasing or decreasing your energy expenditure. Calorie restriction without exercise can even make you "fatter" if you lose more lean mass than fat mass.

Two of the most common goals for improving body composition are losing fat and gaining muscle. If you want to look toned, lean, or strong, then at least one of these goals is yours. If you want to change your shape in any way—rounder glutes, smaller waist, sculpted arms—then at least one of these goals is yours.

But first, let's address the question that many of us have: is it possible to lose fat and gain muscle at the same time? While it is difficult to force both processes to occur, it is possible. Muscles can grow if they are overloaded effectively by using energy from fat stores, but energy from adequate nutrient intake will speed up the process. To lose weight, we need a negative energy balance, and to gain weight, we need a positive energy balance. If we lose fat and gain muscle at the same time, either the processes will occur at such similar rates that we will notice no difference on the scale, or one will have more of an effect on our weight than the other. Our ability to lose fat and gain muscle at the same time is dependent on many factors like genetics and hormones. The easier route is to aim for one of these two goals: aim to lose weight while preserving lean mass, and you will lose fat; aim to gain weight while minimizing fat gain, and you will gain muscle.

To most efficiently lose fat, we must utilize a caloric deficit and resistance training. A caloric deficit ensures that weight is lost, and resistance training ensures that as much muscle is maintained as possible during the weight loss process.

Although we can gain fat cells (adipocytes) when we gain weight, they do not disappear when we lose weight. They just shrink as free fatty acids (FFAs) are released to be used for energy. Hydrolysis splits the triacylglycerol into a glycerol and three fatty acids, and the fat cells release those FFAs into the bloodstream to go where they are needed for energy. The only way to get rid of fat cells is by mechanically removing them, e.g. via liposuction.

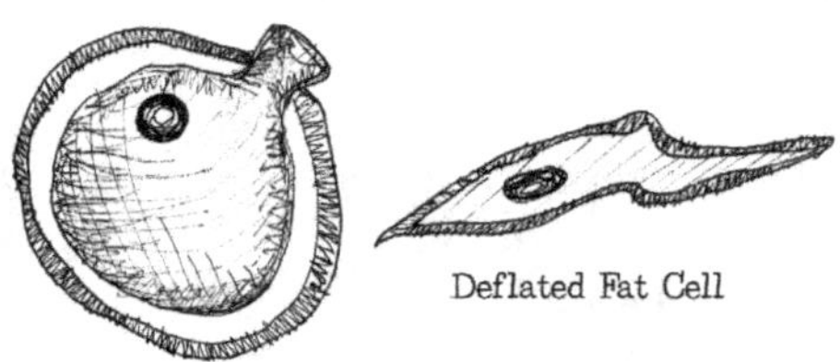
Deflated Fat Cell

Once we start on a fat loss journey, it can become addictive, so try to remember that having some body fat is ideal for overall health. The type and location of fat cells matter too. Hip and butt fat can be protective against certain diseases, at least in females, whereas visceral fat (fat around organs in the abdominal cavity; think of a "beer belly") has immune function and is associated with heightened risk of certain diseases. Unfortunately, we cannot choose where we store and lose fat; genetics decides this for us. This means that "spot reduction" is effectively a myth unless surgery is involved. But don't worry, with hard work, patience, and consistency, fat can be lost from even the most stubborn places.

On the other hand, to gain muscle, we need to eat enough calories and nutrients to rebuild muscle broken down during workouts and to provide energy to be able to complete our workouts. Resistance training causes trauma to muscle fibers, which causes hormones and hormone-like compounds called growth factors to activate satellite cells that repair and form new fibers. In a rested state, the rate of muscle protein breakdown is greater than that of muscle protein synthesis. This means that muscles will atrophy, or shrink, if they are not used. We must work not only to grow muscle but even to maintain our lean mass.

Gaining muscle is typically a much slower process than losing fat. While there are individual differences due to factors like genetics, training history, and severity of caloric surplus, most of us cannot sit around eating ice cream and cookies, even when our goal is to gain weight. In most cases, a slight caloric surplus and resistance training is the best recipe for hypertrophy. Resistance training is necessary for muscle growth; each day of our lives we are effectively losing muscle unless we train them often enough and effectively enough to force muscle maintenance or growth.

Individuals who are new to strength training can train anywhere between one and seven days a week and progress, but more experienced athletes need to train muscles more frequently to continue to overload them. There is a lack of substantial evidence that training too much has negative effects beyond psychological factors and risk of injury. At the same time, rest days are essential for overall physical and mental health. The ideal number of rest days will vary from person to person.

Women can typically recover faster than men and should not fear overtraining. Although women will see faster results when they first start weight training, they will ultimately see slower progress due to hormonal differences. Very muscular, drug-free females (and males!) have spent years or even decades in a caloric surplus trying to gain muscle.

## Self Acceptance

Flexible dieting has become a popular tool to reach very low levels of body fat without destroying one's mental health or overall quality of life. Nevertheless, working to improve one's physique can be a gateway for negative thoughts and behaviors if we are not careful. What are the consequences of being so focused on our physique? Shouldn't we just be happy with ourselves? Indeed, paying attention to our food intake and our body weight and composition can be a tool to either destroy or strengthen self-acceptance. Let's use bodybuilding, which involves focusing on your physique more than anything else, to explore some of the ways in which flexible dieting can improve our self-acceptance.

Bodybuilding is all about "the thrill of the chase." Anyone who has competed in bodybuilding competitions can tell you that the goal each day is to be better than the day before. If you do it right, the focus is on the journey, not an end point.

People who compete in bodybuilding do so for various reasons. Some want to progress further in the sport (e.g. earn professional status and compete as a professional). Some want to prove to themselves or to others that they can set a goal and crush it. Some want to get their name out there and potentially be sponsored by a supplement or apparel company or be recruited for fitness modeling. Everyone has their own personal goals, but regardless of these goals, bodybuilding can be a way for anyone to learn self-acceptance.

This may seem counterintuitive. How can training and preparing for something so superficial teach you how to accept yourself? Bodybuilding is about shredding that final layer of body fat to get to your goal show weight. It is about tweaking your posing just right so you stand out above the rest on stage. How can it be about self-acceptance?

When you are in tune with your body, when you can anticipate how it will respond to a 20 g carbohydrate increase or decrease, then you can achieve greater self-respect. When we have pushed ourselves to our limits and then pushed ourselves even further, we can appreciate what makes us human. We can learn to love ourselves at every stage of the process, every day of our lives.

It will take time. It does not happen overnight. But understanding the steps toward reaching a stage-ready physique and applying them as you see fit to your own life—regardless of whether you ever set foot on that stage—can help you appreciate your own strengths, your uniqueness, your power, your fragility, your body, your mind, and your life.

Flexible dieting can be a fundamental step in the process of self-acceptance by enabling you to take care of your physical and mental health at the same time. Too many fad diets use body shaming as a tool for motivation. Flexible dieting requires an understanding and appreciation of where you are right now as a tool for motivation. Take care of your body and mind now to reap the benefits of maximal progress.

## Make It Your Own

You may have a goal that is not listed here. Nevertheless, flexible dieting can help you live the life you have always imagined for yourself. You may find that this heightened attention to your health will resonate in other areas of your life. Live intentionally. Do good. Feel good. Be good.

Long-term health goals should always come first, but if overall health is under control, you can focus on tweaking your diet, getting adequate exercise and rest, and reducing stress leading up to your next short-term deadline to achieve the best results you possibly can.

# 12
# LONG-TERM SUCCESS

You may have seen extreme weight-loss challenges where people eventually gain back all the weight—or more. Abruptly dropping calories to an extremely low, unsustainable number is a recipe for rebound. The body decreases expenditure in response to decreased intake. To combat this, you can further decrease your caloric intake by eating less or further increase your expenditure through physical activity. You can easily imagine how challenging this can become over time.. A larger starting calorie deficit will give you less room to chip away when you plateau, which may give you less of a chance at long-term success.

Bodyweight regulation favors weight gain, so this process seems like it should be easier in the opposite direction. However, gaining lean mass while minimizing fat gain can be similarly difficult, as we must continue to overload muscles to increase or even maintain muscle size.

Many people think that they are stuck at a certain weight due to genetics. This is not true, but we do each have a biological bodyweight set point, or a weight around which our body seems to function optimally. There is evidence that weight tends to stick around the set point, which often leads to individuals believing that they are forever doomed to stay around a certain weight. So how do we fight to stay away from this number? It comes down to understanding the processes that make weight fluctuations sticky and outsmarting them.

You might go through a time when the process just does not seem to add up. You are in a caloric deficit but you gain weight. Is the energy balance equation screwed up? Was it the gluten-sugar-lactose-saturated, fat-filled food you ate that did it? Does flexible dieting even work?

There is no reason to blame a specific food or event for unintentional weight gain. When things do not go your way, it is usually a sign that calculations are off and you need to tweak your intake or expenditure (or that you need to be patient). It does not mean that the entire system is broken. The superpower of flexible dieting is that it is based on math. And math never gives.

# Consistency

The best diet for you is one to which you can adhere. If you find yourself always going over your calorie intake goals or not quite being able to reach your goals for a specific macronutrient, it might be time to reassess the situation. Do not be afraid to tweak the macronutrient composition so that your diet is working with and not against your lifestyle. This does not mean that you should end up right back where you started, but it could mean swapping 18 g of carbs for 8 g of fat (both 72 calories), for example.

Do not be hard on yourself if you find that you can meet your intake goals most days but go off-track occasionally. Remember that the average intake is what matters. If you can usually meet your macronutrient goals just fine, but you end up way over or under one day, simply adjust the next day (or another day that week), so the average balances out. Let's say you ordered fish and vegetables at a restaurant, and you had no idea they were going to be cooked in oil or butter, so you did not save room for this extra fat in your daily nutrient goals. Simply estimate the amount used, and subtract from your fat the following day. If you calculate something incorrectly, have an emotional eating slip-up and go over your macronutrient goals, or otherwise have a bad day with tracking, just remember that flexible dieting is based on math. You can always add or subtract to make up for something. Most important of all, remember that one meal will not make a difference in the long run. One day will not even make a difference in the long run. The average over time is the key to success.

Remember that calories are king, so if you really mess up and eat way too much fat or cannot get enough fat, for example, that is fine. Just do the math and hit your calories for the day. If you manage to stick to your daily calorie goals despite a slip-up with macronutrients, then adjusting another day's intake is not necessary. Let's pretend you have 0 g fat, 40 g carbohydrates, and 12 g protein left for the day, and you are hungry, but you do not have access to or feel like eating anything with carbohydrates and you have a craving for peanut butter. You might decide to eat two tablespoons of peanut butter right out of the jar instead. That is approximately two hundred calories in either case, so you have reached your calorie goal even though you did not meet your macronutrient goals. Of course, if you do this every day, then you are calorie counting, not tracking macronutrients. If you do this occasionally, and it helps you stay on track, then it is practical flexible dieting.

Slow and steady wins the race. If you put yourself in a steep caloric deficit on day 1, and you are hungry all the time during the first week of your diet, then your diet probably will not last very long. If you are uncomfortably hungry or full all the time, consider tweaking your intake accordingly. If calories are set to lose weight at an appropriate pace and you still feel excessively hungry, make sure your protein and fiber intakes are high enough and that meals are balanced with protein and at least some carbohydrates or fat in each meal. While it is ideal to find out what kind of macronutrient ratio works best for your metabolism and your goals, a high-protein diet with the same overall calories will allow you to progress, regardless of the carbohydrate:fat ratio. Adherence is arguably the most important key to a successful diet. Those of us who continue to chug along at a slow yet consistent pace will outdo the ones who start with excessive, unsustainable calorie and macronutrient objectives.

## Honesty

When weight does not respond to our diet the way we want it to, it can be tempting to fall into denial. "The scale must be broken!" While it is possible for a scale to malfunction, it is more likely that something else caused a weight fluctuation. Hormones; meal timing; water, fiber, and sodium intake; stress; sleep; and inflammation are just some possible causes of temporary weight fluctuations. Variations in these factors are part of normal life, and temporary weight fluctuations are typically no cause for concern. Most of us do not engage in the same activities the exact same way every day.

Do not confuse bloating with fat gain. Specific foods can also trigger bloating and temporary weight gain (but not fat gain) in certain individuals, particularly those with irritable bowel syndrome (IBS) and other digestive disorders. Short-chain carbohydrates and sugar alcohols collectively known as FODMAPs (fermentable, oligo-, di-, monosaccharides, and polyols)—fructose (when in excess of glucose), fructans, galactooligosaccharides (GOS), lactose, and polyols (e.g. sorbitol and mannitol)—are either poorly absorbed or not at all. FODMAPs pull water into the small intestine and are fermented by gut bacteria. Next, they generate gases in the large intestine. The result is an increased volume of intestinal contents and discomfort associated with bloating. While you might want to avoid high quantities of FODMAPs if they give you discomfort and bloating, bloating-related weight gain from FODMAPs should not be confused with fat gain.

Even if you eat the same foods every day at the same times, your weigh-ins will be affected by other variables, such as hormonal fluctuations depending on which phase of dieting (or not dieting) you are in, menstrual cycles in females, and a wide variety of other factors, such as antibiotics. It is impossible to control for all factors. Remember that flexible dieting can outsmart these internal regulation mechanisms, but we should also do what we can to optimize these processes to make it easier on ourselves.

While weight is affected by several factors, like poop, food, and water, it is still the one of the best markers of progress that we have, along with body measurements and progress pictures. The other options, like energy, strength, and hunger levels are subjective. Even body measurements and body fat measurements are prone to error.

To minimize error with weight, always check your weight in the morning when you first wake up (preferably around the same time every day) with the same scale. You can either weigh yourself every day and compare weekly averages or weigh yourself only once a week. While weighing yourself daily may be a more accurate method, it can also lead to an unhealthy obsession about weight. A common strategy is to check weight once a week upon waking (with the same scale). Combined with body measurements or even a subjective comparison of how clothes fit or how progress pictures are looking, this can be an extremely effective method.

Whether you are working with a professional or someone else to hold you accountable or doing this on your own, avoid trying to rationalize weight fluctuations too much. Although you should try to understand why your body might act a certain way, resisting or making a change because of speculation can be problematic. "I just need to poop" or "I didn't get enough sleep" or "I must have had too much sodium" or "I didn't drink enough water" or "It's that time of the month" all describe contributing factors to temporary weight fluctuations, but none of them provide measurable data. Do not act on assumptions; act on observations.

It is natural to want to assign blame for our plateaus or rebounds, but at the end of the day, doing so will not get us any closer to our goals. Life is not a lab, and we cannot possibly keep track of all variables that are always at play. The good news is that tracking all variables is not necessary with a flexible dieting approach. The idea is to let life continue normally while we keep track of our dietary intake and weight. We will never be exact, but we do not have to be exact to make progress. We just need to be honest.

Even if you do your best to track everything, it is inevitable that you will run into incorrect reporting, for example, by making mistakes weighing food, not finishing meals, or sneaking extra bites. If you continue to cut or increase calories and do not see results, check to see if there are any areas where you can improve. Self-reporting will always be prone to error. Just remember that keeping your approach as honest as possible will give you the best understanding and lead to the best results.

We must learn to see our ourselves as objectively as possible to maximize success with flexible dieting. We tend to be too hard on ourselves. This is where having a coach or someone else to just take another look at your current situation can be critical to long-term success. Unfortunately, we tend to distort reality when we see ourselves in the mirror. Competitors preparing for bodybuilding competitions tend to think they have much less weight to lose than they really do. Individuals aspiring to look like fitness models often forget that eating enough to gain lean mass is critical to attaining a muscular, toned physique. Perfectionists will always see something else that can be improved. If you feel like nothing you do with your nutrition or exercise is ever enough, talk to someone about it.

Flexible dieting is a way to take care of ourselves, not hurt ourselves. Check in with yourself every so often to make sure that you are in fact taking care of yourself. If you feel down about any part of the process, reach out to a family member, friend, coach, or professional.


## Hormones

The two main appetite hormones are leptin and ghrelin. Leptin is known as "the satiety hormone" for its role in inhibiting hunger. Leptin helps to regulate body weight by decreasing when we lose fat and increasing when we gain fat. In contrast to leptin, ghrelin, the "hunger hormone," sends signal to the brain when it is time to eat. Ghrelin increases in response to fasting or decreased caloric intake.

Cortisol, the stress hormone, increases in a caloric deficit. When carbohydrate intake or overall calorie intake is very low, cortisol can trigger the expression of enzymes needed to break down protein into amino acids and generate glucose from the amino acids and other substrates (glycerol, lactate) in a process known as gluconeogenesis. Avoiding extremely low calorie diets can help to prevent unnecessary cortisol increases.

Both males and females require a normal balance of sex hormones (androgens, estrogens, and progestogens) to maintain normal body functions. Dieting decreases testosterone levels, which can result in fatigue, slowed fat loss, muscle loss, and low sex drive. Adequate rest and recovery, appropriate strength training, and the diet strategies explained in the next section can help combat the decrease in testosterone that comes with dieting. Hormonal disruption from low carbohydrates or low total calories can cause hypothalamic amenorrhea in women, which is a stop or disruption of the menstrual cycle in response to starvation or stress. As a result, women can suffer from low levels of estrogen, progesterone, testosterone, luteinizing hormone (LH), and follicle-stimulating hormone (FSH). To optimize hormone levels when dieting and minimize negative side effects, caloric intake should be kept sufficiently high to avoid these conditions.

## Breaking through Plateaus

While starvation mode is effectively a myth, our Total Daily Energy Expenditure (TDEE) does adjust as our body weight and composition change. Plateaus are inevitable unless we continually change our diet to account for changes in energy expenditure. A common mistake for many new dieters is to calculate an appropriate caloric or macronutrient intake to start making progress and never change it. It is not a good idea to stick to the same macronutrient intake goals for the duration of your diet, "bulk," or even maintenance phase. Your energy expenditure changes as your weight and body composition change. We tend to decrease our overall activity level when metabolic rate decreases, which further decreases energy expenditure. It is therefore important to either recalculate or simply adjust your intake based on changes in body weight and composition.

Many of the body's adaptations to dieting are collectively known as adaptive thermogenesis. Metabolic rate decreases, but the purpose of adjusting your macronutrient intake goals is not to account for changes in BMR. Your BMR changes extremely slowly since the only variable likely changing is weight. Age, height, and gender take much more time to change. So while your body burns less energy at rest (resting energy expenditure or REE) as you lose weight, non-resting energy expenditure (NREE) may decrease at a much more notable rate. You burn less energy during exercise (exercise activity thermogenesis or EAT) and through non-exercise activity thermogenesis (NEAT). The thermic effect of food (TEF) also decreases. While these changes are expected when dieting, they are not always predictable.

NEAT can account for large discrepancies in our daily energy expenditure. Fidgety people tend to burn more calories than people who stand still simply from fidgeting more. For many of us, NEAT decreases when dieting; we feel sluggish and tired from eating less, so our bodies react by expending less energy. Some individuals may experience a phenomenon where they keep increasing cardio, but their bodies adjust by decreasing NEAT, so they are not increasing expenditure as much as they think. Your entire lifestyle—not just your exercise time—contributes to your energy expenditure. When we gain weight, our bodies may react by increasing or decreasing NEAT; a caloric surplus makes some feel energized and others feel sluggish. We can intentionally increase NEAT by walking more, standing instead of sitting, taking the stairs, dancing, laughing, etc. Many of us have jobs where we sit for hours and hours. Get up and move to increase NEAT.

## Components of Energy Expenditure

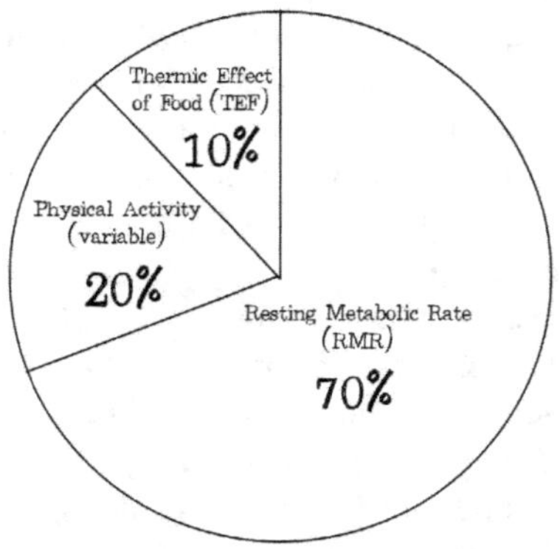


As TDEE decreases, either food needs to be lowered or exercise needs to be increased to get TDEE back up. Someone trying to lose weight without doing any exercise would have to continually lower intake until he or she is consuming very little because there is no physical activity to increase the expenditure side of the equation. On the other hand, if the goal is gaining weight, then TDEE will increase as weight is gained, so you will need to keep adding food or cutting back on activity.

While these adaptations cause plateaus during dieting that are not very fun, there is at least anecdotal evidence that we can adjust to caloric intake in the other direction too. The process of progressively increasing calories while gaining as little weight as possible is sometimes referred to as "reverse dieting" in the bodybuilding industry. The idea is that instead of knocking off calories when your weight plateaus, we can stack them back on. The speed at which you add on calories will depend on your specific metabolism (e.g. how quickly your body adjusts to the caloric changes) and goals (i.e. how fast do you want to pack on the weight?).

While increasing caloric intake does very gradually increase metabolic rate as weight increases and hormone levels increase, there is no magic to "reverse dieting" that allows us to maintain or even lose weight while eating more. Increasing energy intake can simply make us expend more energy. If you just dieted for six months and I tell you to increase your carbohydrate intake by a mere 10 g of carbs this week, you might think, "Wow, I have all this new energy." Maybe you kill your workouts; maybe you simply start moving more. Your body might even respond by revving up the internal regulation to increase NREE. On the other hand, maybe none of these things occur, and you gain weight. Reverse dieting is not magic; bodyweight regulation just occurs in both directions—plus there's a placebo effect of thinking you have all this new energy and motivation.

Let's get back to dieting for a minute. We must continually increase expenditure or decrease intake when we plateau in a caloric deficit. Simultaneously, our appetite hormones adjust so that we feel hungrier and more tired when we diet. The good news is that you can ease the pains of dieting by distributing your caloric intake over the course of the week in such a way that works best for your lifestyle.

Let's discuss some specific approaches to manipulating caloric intake.

## Calorie Cycling

Some people prefer to adhere to different calorie and macronutrient intake goals on training days and rest days, or more active days and less active days. This is a great idea if your workouts are extremely intense and your rest days are extremely sedentary. If you like to keep active all days, then different macronutrient intake goals for different days of the week is likely not necessary. On the other hand, some prefer to utilize calorie cycling because they can stick their diet better. For example, it can be easier to stick to lower calories for a few days if you know that you will get higher calories later in the week rather than being stuck at relatively low calories for a seemingly endless period.

Adjusting your dietary intake based on the intensity of your workouts is dangerous when it verges on a free for all. For example, if your workout was extra intense or long today, or if you walked an extra five miles today, then it makes sense to add more food, right? The problem is that we can easily make excuses on any given day for why we "need" to increase or decrease calories. It is not inherently problematic to calorie cycle, but we just need to make sure the cycling is structural. Otherwise we defeat the purpose of having set goals. When the guidelines are so blurred that you can't see them anymore, we are no longer flexible dieting. At that point, we have crossed the line into more of an intuitive eating approach. There's nothing wrong with that. It is just not flexible dieting.

Calorie cycling can be adapted to fit your preferences and lifestyle. Remember that the weekly average is more important than any given day, so even if your energy balance equation is tipped in the wrong direction one day, as long as it tips back in the right direction when you look at the overall average, you will progress.


## Intermittent Fasting (IF)

Intermittent fasting (IF) is a form of calorie cycling where dietary intake is set to zero or a very small number of calories for a certain period. By greatly reducing calories for certain days or time periods, IF allows for higher-calorie days or time periods when fasting is not scheduled. Two popular approaches to IF that have been studied are (1) feasting and fasting times and (2) the 5:2 approach. The first involves fasting for a certain amount of time every day, and the second involves fasting for two whole days out of the week.

It takes several hours to deplete glycogen that is stored in the liver after eating; after that, the body will start burning fat. A feasting window of several hours therefore gives enough time for this process to occur; however, there are benefits to even longer feasting windows. Instead of trying to spread out a caloric deficit so that it lasts from the time you wake up until the time to go to sleep and suffering from hunger pangs when you run out of food, a shorter window of eating time allows for bigger meals and less hunger during the feasting window. On the other hand, you might find that you feel too hungry during the fasting window and prefer to spread out the calories. IF can be similarly useful in a caloric surplus. Some people find it annoying to be constantly eating; others prefer to spread out the calories.

The 5:2 fasting approach to dieting is more extreme. It involves five days at maintenance calories and two days at five hundred calories (or whatever deficit you decide to use). This is a great option because your body only knows you're dieting two days out of the week; however, it is not the best fit for everyone.

## Carb Cycling

Carbohydrate cycling ("carb cycling") is a specific type of calorie cycling in which caloric intake is arranged so that there are higher-carbohydrate and lower-carbohydrate days throughout the week. Carbohydrates provide quick energy and can affect levels of insulin and leptin, among other key players in our internal regulation processes. There is no "best practice" for implementing carb cycling. You may need to experiment to see what works best for your lifestyle. Small adjustments can be made to protein and fat according to personal metabolism and preference.

Carb cycling can be especially useful when overall carbohydrate intake is very low. As with general calorie cycling, for some people it is easier to suffer through a few carb-free or low-carb days if they get to have some medium-carb days rather than all very-low-carb days. For example, three days at 30 g carbohydrates and one day at 100 g carbohydrates might not sound as scary as four days at 47.5 g carbohydrates. On the other hand, some might want to take a more moderate approach rather than suffering through those low-carb days.

## Refeeds

A refeed is a type of carb cycling in which one high-carbohydrate day is taken or multiple high-carbohydrate days are taken consecutively. Increasing carbohydrate intake can increase leptin and insulin levels and energy expenditure. Since menstruation can cease when leptin levels are low enough, refeed days can be especially critical for women who are dieting for a long time. Insulin inhibits muscle protein breakdown and can stimulate testosterone production, so boosting insulin can also help to reduce some unwanted physiological adaptations to dieting.

The frequency of refeed days and the percentage increase in carbohydrates necessary on refeed days depend on numerous factors including length of diet, how severe the calorie deficit is, carbohydrate intake, body fat level, physical activity level, and genetics. Generally, the more you normally restrict your carbohydrate intake, the more carbohydrates you will need to consume for a refeed.

Because one of the main purposes of a refeed day is to increase glycogen stores, many people opt for starchy carbohydrate sources rather than fructose-heavy sources. This is fine, but just keep in mind that the overall picture of the diet is what matters. Avoiding fructose entirely on refeed days means avoiding fruit. Eating a banana with your breakfast is not the same as getting all your carbohydrates for the day from bananas.

One of the main benefits of implementing refeed days is the psychological impact. Remember that adherence is a key predictor for success.

## Diet Breaks

Unlike calorie cycling, a diet break is, as its name suggests, a complete break from your diet. Usually a "diet break" refers to a period of days or weeks (often one or two weeks). The idea is to allow enough time for leptin and thyroid hormone to increase back to more normal levels. During the diet break, caloric intake should be raised to approximately maintenance level. It is a good idea to be conservative when you set these maintenance calories, since the caloric intake needed to maintain your weight after dieting for some time will be lower than what it was before you started dieting.

To estimate your new maintenance calories, start by taking your average daily calories consumed over past week or month. Then take the weight you have lost over same time and divide as necessary to find average weight lost per week. If you lost four pounds last month, you lost an average of one pound per week. Multiply whatever number you get by five hundred. For our example, we have $1 \times 500 = 500$ calories. Then you add this number to the daily average calories consumed to estimate your current maintenance intake.

Some people prefer not to track their intake during a diet break, which can lead to unnecessary fat gain if eating gets out of control or even a continuation in a caloric deficit if eating is kept too restricted. As with any phase of the dieting process, it is optimal to give yourself at least a range of calorie and macronutrient intake goals. For example, aim for 250–260 g carbohydrates per day.

You can expect to maintain your weight on a diet break if you do it correctly. However, some might gain weight, and some might even lose weight on a diet break. In either case, some of the weight lost or gained could be water weight. If you lose weight, the part that is not water weight could in fact be fat loss due to increased intake allowing for increased expenditure, thereby tipping the energy balance equation back in the weight loss direction.

Some people also take breaks from the process of gaining weight; these are typically called "mini cuts." As with diet breaks, the idea is to give yourself a break from the psychological and physiological effects of changing your body weight and body composition. If you stay in a caloric surplus too long, you might start to gain more fat than you would like. On the other hand, you just might be sick of eating so much. You can use the same approach as above to estimate your current maintenance caloric intake, but subtract the final number from your current daily average calories consumed instead of adding. From there, you can continue to decrease calories to encourage weight loss at your desired pace. A break from gaining weight is typically longer than a diet break, as the goal is to lose some fat and not just give your body a chance to recoup.

While there can be physiological benefits to taking breaks, sometimes you need to take a break from dieting or gaining weight just to give yourself a mental break.

## Untracked Meals

Tracking dietary intake all the time can get tiring. An occasional untracked meal allows for a mental break and renewed focus when you get back to tracking. Individuals who take untracked meals typically follow their normal mealtime macronutrient goals during the entire day except for the one meal that they choose to be a free meal. This can be done as often as is desired. Just keep in mind that the purpose of flexible dieting is to provide external regulation since many of us cannot logically regulate our own dietary intake. If your approach is always flexible and you are used to estimating portions, then an untracked meal can give you an opportunity to forget about numbers and hopefully eat more than what your diet allows. However, free meals can be problematic if you usually track your macronutrient intake to the exact gram and use the lack of rigidity as an excuse to either go overboard and binge or to continue to restrict and even undereat during the untracked meal. Despite its potential for disaster, a free meal can be just enough to refuel and get you feeling ready to get back on track with flexible dieting when the meal is over.

Even if you are the most meticulous, careful, strong-minded individual, dieting can warp your thought process. An untracked meal can easily turn into such a high-calorie meal that your daily average for the week pushes out of a caloric deficit and into a caloric surplus. Burgers with fries, whole pizzas, or large hot-fudge sundaes can creep up to 2,000+ calories each, so be mindful if you do decide to implement untracked meals. Calories still count even if we choose not to track them.

## Moderation is Key

As you focus on reaching your goals, always keep in mind that moderation is key. We discussed hormonal changes when dieting. Remember that these changes can make us want to eat more than we need to reach our goals. Our bodies have evolved to store fat.

One common excuse when "cheating" on our diet is, "I went off a little, so I just decided to throw the whole day and start again tomorrow." For example, "I had one Oreo, so I just ate all of them," or "I splurged at dinner, so I got dessert too." These habits are extremely detrimental because you end up much farther away from your goal than if you just accepted the initial mistake and moved on. Throwing the whole day or meal is like saying, "I spent five dollars over budget, so I went ahead and spent five hundred dollars over." It makes no sense.

So what should you do if you splurge a little? You can either adjust another day as previously discussed so the weekly average is virtually unaffected, or you can simply ignore the hiccup and continue as planned. One day won't make a difference in the long run, but if you make it a habit of letting things slide, then one day can add up to weeks or even months. For many of us, the best approach is to accept the mistake and move on as normal.

The trick with moderation is to find the best approach for you and stick to it. Remember that consistency is the only way to make progress. Some people can eat one Girl Scout cookie every day and be satisfied and motivated by getting to have their treat the following day. Others will feel the need to continue eating cookies, leading to an unplanned caloric surplus, which can be dangerous. These individuals might be able to work toward a more balanced approach, but for anyone in a steep caloric deficit or who has been dieting for a long time, sweets or "junk food" can be a slippery slope. Highly palatable foods tempt the taste buds and are low in volume, so they do not fill the stomach or provide satiety after eating. Many individuals do well consuming a high-volume meal, for example, lean protein with both fibrous and starchy vegetables, and following it up with a small treat, like a Hershey's kiss. Food should satiate your stomach and mind. There is room for small treats if you feel comfortable allowing them. If not, that's fine too.

## When and How to Stop Dieting

After spending months in a caloric deficit with a decreasing metabolic rate and changing hormone levels, there comes a time when enough is enough. It might happen before you reach your goal weight, but you can always come back to dieting and push farther after taking some time off if that happens. So how do you know when the diet is over? And what can we do to prevent rebound?

Is it time to consider ending your diet if you are hungry all the time and craving foods you never thought you would crave? Not necessarily. In fact, these are often just signs that you are dieting, not signs that you need to stop dieting. There are both psychological and physiological reasons to stop dieting. When the hunger and cravings are all you can think about, when you are unable to address other issues in your everyday life, it might be time to stop dieting. When your body weight and composition are not responding to decreases in your dietary intake or increases in your energy expenditure, it might be time to stop dieting. When deciding whether you are ready to stop dieting, keep in mind that it is all relative. One person might be comfortable dieting to less than 10% body fat while someone else might feel that the measures necessary to get there are compromising his or her quality of life. If you find no happiness in your diet, it is time to get out. Above all else, assure that you want to do what you are doing.

To stop your diet, you should not return to your normal lifestyle as it was before you entered a caloric deficit. This is a recipe for rebound. A structured diet deserves a structured exit. So how do we ease out? There are several approaches. A diet break as described earlier could be enough for you, but realistically we need longer than a couple of weeks at maintenance before we can safely start a new diet. Calories can be eased back up slowly or quickly. As mentioned earlier, a slow increase in calories is sometimes called a reverse diet. While dieting requires continually decreasing calories, reverse dieting requires continually increasing calories. This way, we can prevent rapid, immediate excess fat gain. However, many prefer to increase calories quicker because slowly increasing calories can result in intense hunger and a painfully slow return of hormones to baseline levels. Regardless of the speed at which you increase the calories, the purpose is to give your body a chance to normalize before you continue to push it beyond its limits or to focus on maintaining your current physique. Many people take this time to focus on gaining muscle to improve their shape and body composition.

If you were consuming 3,000 calories per day before you started dieting, and you were maintaining your weight, that does not mean you can return to 3,000 calories and maintain weight when your diet is over. Because of all the physiological adaptations to dieting, including a new, lower body weight, your new maintenance intake will be much lower than it was before your diet. Increasing calories too quickly can cause unwanted fat gain, but keeping yourself in a caloric deficit for too long can unnecessarily prolong the negative effects of dieting. A structured exit from a diet involves finding your new maintenance as quickly as possible and slowly increasing calories to a surplus to minimize fat gain while allowing your body to get back up to healthy state. I like to call this process a structured exit, but in the bodybuilding community, this process is often called a "reverse diet" or a "lean bulk."

The concept of a reverse diet is rather controversial in the bodybuilding community. To some, reverse dieting describes a process through which you increase calories so subtly that you remain in a caloric deficit for weeks or months before even approaching your new maintenance calories let alone gaining any weight. However, research suggests that the metabolic adaptations to dieting go away after returning to maintenance, even without a structured exit, so there is no long-term harm in slowly increasing calories after a diet. The main benefit of increasing calories so slowly after a diet is simply that you can eat more food while maintaining or improving your body composition and maintaining or decreasing your body weight. It may sound vain, but for someone who mentally cannot handle the idea of gaining weight or fat, the best thing might be eating more food to start the recovery process.

Many claim that a slow increase in calories after dieting is a waste of time because our body can overcome adaptations on its own; however, the capacity for metabolic rate to change can vary from individual to individual. Additionally, some individuals might not be mentally prepared to start gaining fat after a diet. In 2014, my daily caloric intake increased over five months from 1,440 to 2,195.5. I went from doing five sessions of 30 minutes of cardio per week to doing no cardio. My macronutrient intake went from 29 g fat, 135 g carbohydrates, and 160 g protein to 59.5 g fat, 255 g carbohydrates, and 160 g protein. Over those five months, my weight actually decreased from 120 lb to 118 lb. It is likely that I would have gained weight if I had made these changes over a shorter period. This type of slow, structured exit may work well for individuals who have been in a caloric deficit for a very long time or who are not mentally prepared to gain weight after a diet.

It is not uncommon to lose weight or appear leaner when you begin a slow, structured exit from a diet. Note that this does not mean the system is broken. You have not found a way to change science. Remember we talked about outsmarting the system, not being able to change it altogether. What is likely happening in these cases is that hormones start to return to normal levels, and energy expenditure increases faster than we are increasing intake. More food means more intense workouts, which means more calories burned. As with dieting, we can tweak the pace of a structured exit from a diet to fit your specific goals and situation. Someone who has dieted for a bodybuilding competition and is suffering from brain fog, low testosterone, and other negative health effects may need to increase calories much faster than someone who is just tired of dieting.

## Stay Motivated

Before you try any techniques to break through plateaus, the first necessary step is optimizing your mindset. You must tell yourself that you are able to outsmart these adaptations and that you are willing to power through. It is easy to make excuses for ourselves about why we cannot accomplish our goals. Slow metabolism, fast metabolism, bone structure, body shape, no time—the excuses go on and on.

If you can look at someone else's accomplishments and say, "I could never do that," then the motivation is not there. The difference between one who achieves and one who does not is not that one had an easier time or better luck, but rather that one said, "I can." Once you understand that you can unlock your potential, all it takes to fulfill that potential is one step in the right direction. We are the result of one of an infinite number of possible outcomes. Look toward the end of your desired path, envision the potential you that you want to become, and proceed in that direction.

If you love the outcome you see at the end of the path but cannot find happiness along the path, then you will not make it to the end. You must find happiness in the journey, comfort in the uncomfortable, and purpose in the struggle. To keep your momentum and continue success over a long period of time, instead of making excuses and complaining, try articulating what you want and how you are going to get there. Check to make sure you always have a SMART goal that you will be able to check off and add to the pile when you complete it.

Do not let yourself get discouraged by speed bumps. If you know you made a mistake, acknowledge it and move on. On the other hand, if you know you are doing everything you should be doing, and you are not seeing progress, take a step back to assess the situation. If you are seeing progress in the wrong direction, it's time to reevaluate your method and make sure there are no errors. But if you have simply hit a plateau, or your weight moved in the wrong direction for a few days, give your body a chance to regroup before giving up or being hard on yourself. You can do this!

# 13

# POWDERS AND PILLS

The dietary supplement industry, worth billions and billions of dollars, encompasses various powders, pills, bars, and liquid versions of vitamins, minerals, "botanical" or herbal products, amino acid products, and enzyme products. As per the FDA website, the "FDA is not authorized to review dietary supplement products for safety and effectiveness before they are marketed."

Supplements are ancillary to your diet; supplements are not food. They can contribute to a very small percentage of your success. Additionally, research often suggests that extracted nutrients in the form of many dietary supplements may not have all the positive benefits that whole foods can have.

For healthy individuals (i.e. individuals with no major diagnoses or issues) who are trying to maintain or gain weight, it is unlikely that nutrient supplementation is necessary if diet composition is balanced and varied. This is where meal plans that have you consuming the exact same meal every day can fall short. When we eat the same foods every day, it is likely that we will end up with inadequate intake of certain nutrients and excess intake of others.

For healthy individuals who are trying to lose weight, it is important to take their personal situation into account when deciding whether supplements are necessary. Someone in a slight caloric deficit may be able to get adequate nutrients, while someone in a steep caloric deficit looking to cut a large amount of weight before a specific event may find it difficult to get adequate nutrients from food alone. For instance, when calories are too low or even when carbohydrates are too low despite a reasonably high caloric intake, it can be difficult to get enough fiber. In these cases, a fiber supplement can be useful to encourage healthy digestion and bowel movements. Additionally, regardless of whether you are dieting, if you are performing intense workouts or otherwise very active, you may need to supplement with electrolytes or other nutrients to aid in recovery.

If you choose to use supplements, it is wise to do so under the supervision of a healthcare professional.

## Safety and Regulation

In 2015, New York Attorney General Eric Schneiderman announced that studies conducted by his office found that four out of five herbal supplements tested at GNC, Target, Wal-Mart, and Walgreens in New York did not contain the ingredients stated on the label and that over a third of them contained "contaminants." Others posited that these tests were unreliable and that these products did indeed contain what was listed on their ingredient lists. Regardless of who was right and who was wrong, the importance of the issue is that we as consumers cannot be confident about the contents contained within these powders and pills. Most of us do not have the resources to test products that we buy to determine the actual ingredients.

Supplements have been recalled for harmful or potentially harmful effects due to contamination by microorganisms, pesticides, heavy metals, and other substances; an ingredient claimed to be in the product is not actually in it; an ingredient claimed to be in the product in a certain amount is in the product but in a different amount. These are all risks to keep in mind when buying supplements. Even if supplement ingredients have been shown to be effective, the possibility for contamination and untruthful labeling makes it difficult to know just how effective a supplement will be.

Sometimes when we cannot get results through Western medicine, we resort to the mysterious, promising world of supplements. Often without any prescription from a health professional, we do our own research and purchase products that offer a chance at improved health, sometimes even when we have no real health problem. Despite our incredible human capacity to meet our fitness and health goals through hard work and consistency alone, supplements remain incredibly popular.

## Multivitamins

When you hear "vitamin," you might think of a pill, but vitamins and minerals are organic compounds found in foods. We know that many vitamins and minerals aid in essential body functions, but we also know that food is the best source of vitamins, minerals, and other beneficial compounds. Yet, we isolate these compounds and put them in pills in extremely high doses. Foods have exactly what we need, if only we were to eat nutrient-dense foods in appropriate amounts.

While we can get all vitamins and minerals through food, if you have a restrictive diet, lack access to a variety of foods, or have high risk factors or a specific heath situation that requires a large quantity of a specific micronutrient, then a trustworthy supplement might in fact be useful for you. Except for vitamin D, most of us can reach all our micronutrient needs through food alone. And we can spend time outside to get extra vitamin D.

Excess vitamin intake can be not only unnecessary but even harmful. While excess water-soluble vitamins are excreted in urine, excess fat-soluble vitamins can be stored. On one hand, this means that children who have night blindness and other symptoms of vitamin A deficiency can be rid of symptoms for six months after only one pill. However, in America, vitamin A deficiency is extremely rare. Moreover, treatment of disease with fat-soluble vitamins such as vitamin A and vitamin E may be associated with increased mortality. The main takeaway relative to vitamin supplements is to remember that more is not always better.

## Diet Pills

Common types of weight loss supplements include: appetite suppressants, which are supposed to decrease appetite and desire to eat; fat burners, which are supposed to help the burn body fat; and calorie blockers, which are supposed to block the absorption of fats or carbohydrates.

Many appetite suppressants are not backed by substantial evidence. Ginger and 5-HTP, the precursor of serotonin, are examples of supplements commonly used for suppressing appetite. Adrenaline is an appetite suppressant, so drinking coffee or trying a new, exciting activity or workout may suppress appetite.

Caffeine is one of the most popular and effective fat-burning supplements. Caffeine does in fact stimulate metabolic rate, and taking caffeine at multiple times throughout the day can prolong its effects, although insomnia is not an uncommon side effect. Caffeine may also increase strength performance if taken before a workout. Just be aware that individual responses to caffeine can vary. As a central nervous system stimulant, caffeine can cause harmful side effects in high doses. The tolerable dose will vary among individuals. We can also develop a tolerance to caffeine over time, which means that we need to consume more of it to have the same effect. For this reason, it is wise to consume caffeine in small doses and to take occasional breaks if you do choose to consume it.

Other fat burners include capsaicin, clenbuterol (illegal), ephedrine, 7-keto DHEA, nicotine, and yohimbine. Fat burners can interfere with medications and other supplements, so the advice of a healthcare professional is highly recommended.

Calorie blockers are meant to block carbohydrate or fat-digesting enzymes from either being released from the pancreas or from acting on their substrates. Calorie blockers can cause digestive issues and are not as effective as many think. Instead of using these supplements as an excuse to overeat, we should just avoid overeating.

A safer approach to losing weight is to increase activity level and/or decrease food intake.

## Protein Powders, Bars, and Ready-to-Drink Products

Protein powder is used by gym-goers because of its convenience, sweet taste, and fast delivery of nutrients. Whey protein is known to be a great post-workout option because of its quick absorption, but any powder will absorb faster than most foods. The same thing happens with foods blended into a smoothie or shake; the smaller particles will be absorbed quicker because they do not need to be broken down like a whole fruit does, for example. Similarly, blended oats have a higher GI than whole oats; they are absorbed quicker and therefore quickly raise blood glucose and insulin levels.

If you want the quickest digestion and absorption, hydrolyzed whey isolate, formed by splitting proteins into amino acids, may be your best bet. Other protein powders, regardless of whether they are isolates (meaning their content is at least 90% protein), are made of larger peptide structures.

Protein bars and ready-to-drink supplements typically have some form of protein powder as an ingredient. These supplements can be convenient ways to reach your nutrition goals, but often the quality of ingredients and truthfulness behind the labels are unknown. Just remember that supplements are supplementary; they are not dietary staples.

## Popular Sports Supplements

Pre-workout, intra-workout, post-workout, morning, nighttime, with meals, in between meals—there are products advertised to help you reach your fitness goals for any time of the day or night. When we buy supplements with long lists of ingredients or proprietary blends, it is critical that we research and understand exactly what we are going to be putting into our bodies. Check the amount of each ingredient listed; do they match what research shows are efficacious doses? Does the caffeine content exceed what you know you can handle? Sometimes these products are recalled due to dangerous findings, so investigate before throwing your money at these companies. What follows is a list of some commonly used sports nutrition supplements that have been selected based on how frequently they are advertised and used—not how effective they actually are.

## Electrolytes

For the most part, we can get all the nutrients we need from food, although certain sports supplements can be beneficial for athlete. Taking electrolyte supplements or consuming foods high in electrolytes is critical for athletes. Be aware that some of these supplements have added sugar and may or may not make sense to consume with your nutrient intake goals.

## Amino Acids

Branched-chain amino acids (BCAAs), leucine, isoleucine, and valine are purported to help with muscle hypertrophy and endurance. There is evidence that consumption of leucine in a fasted state can improve muscle protein synthesis. If you are fasting for some reason, BCAAs might be beneficial. Otherwise, focusing on getting adequate protein through your diet is probably a better use of your time.

## Creatine Monohydrate

Creatine monohydrate is arguably the best supplement for improving strength. It also increases intramuscular hydration. Other types of creatine supplements and creatine blends can be unnecessarily expensive and less effectively absorbed. Appropriate creatine dosing may depend on body weight, muscle mass, and activity level.

## Beta-alanine

Beta-alanine can increase muscle carnosine levels and delay lactic acid buildup, which may increase the amount of high-intensity work that you can perform. A common side effect of beta-alanine is a tingly feeling called paresthesia. A standard dose is 2–5 g, but taking smaller doses will help to avoid paresthesia.

## Citrulline

Citrulline is an amino acid that is part of the urea cycle. It may decrease fatigue and soreness. Eight grams of citrulline malate has been shown to increase maximal grip strength, lower body explosive power, and number of repetitions of lower body exercises performed before reaching failure. Some people take L-arginine to increase nitric oxide in the body, but citrulline may increase plasma arginine levels more effectively than arginine.

## Glutamine

Glutamine is an essential amino acid found in muscle tissue. Many people think glutamine will help them with muscle growth or soreness after workouts, but the intestines absorb glutamine and only a small amount makes it to the muscles. Glutamine is therefore a better supplement for digestive health than for muscle growth.

## Testosterone Boosters

If you have low testosterone, then correcting this with a prescription from a doctor can make a big difference in your life, but if you have normal testosterone levels, you probably do not need a testosterone-boosting supplement, nor will you see a big difference if you take one.

Of course, if you have the money, you can buy whatever supplements you want, but strength training, eating enough, and sleeping enough are far more critical to physique and performance goals.

## Proceed with Caution

There are thousands of other supplements in addition to those listed in this book. When we consume "health supplements," we reap the benefits of believing that we are doing something healthy, which could have a nice placebo effect and perhaps even encourage us to make more healthy decisions.

Just as the goal is not to obsess about food during every waking hour, the goal is not to obsess over which powders and pills will maximize your results. If you stick to your daily nutrient intake goals and consistently tweak them when progress stalls, you will get the results you want, regardless of which supplements you are or are not taking.

Extremely high doses of single nutrients can have harmful effects. Just because a compound occurs naturally in food does not mean that it is effective, necessary, or safe to take as a supplement.

Supplement interactions with conventional drugs are not fully understood, so it is common for surgeons to ask their patients to stop taking them prior to undergoing medical procedures.

# 14
# ALTERNATIVE APPROACHES

Flexible dieting is undoubtedly one approach that can help you reach your goals, but is it the right approach for you?

One of the main benefits of flexible dieting is that you can reach your goals without having to change your lifestyle. It sounds like it is too good to be true, but as we have discussed, flexible dieting merely requires doing some math (or eyeballing portions if you do not want to commit to doing the math). You just have to take the appropriate portions of whatever is available to you and fit it into the outline of the nutrient requirements that are appropriate for you based on your situation and goals. Flexible dieting is no more than a fundamental awareness of what you eat and why you eat it.

However, there are disadvantages to a flexible dieting approach. First of all, once you see foods as their macronutrient and micronutrient components, you cannot unsee them in that way. A candy bar that you once enjoyed is now a dose of carbohydrates and fat. For individuals who have a history of obsessing over food in a way that negatively impacts upon their lives, tracking dietary intake might be a poor long-term approach. At the same time, many health professionals will request such individuals to track their dietary intake upon seeking treatment. Aside from potentially triggering negative thoughts or behaviors, flexible dieting requires an attention to detail that you may simply not want to bother with.

If you have decided that flexible dieting is not a good fit for you, consider why it is not the best fit. Is it because you are not interested in tracking your intake? Are you susceptible to obsessing over food and do not want to risk a balanced approach taking an unhealthy turn?

## Intuitive Eating

If you do not want to track your intake, a more "intuitive" approach might be right for you. Like flexible dieting, intuitive eating requires an understanding of how food will impact your health. However, unlike flexible dieting, intuitive eating depends on listening to hunger cues instead of tracking numbers. The general idea is to eat when you are hungry and stop when you are full, to always eat with mindfulness and awareness.

Mindful eating is like intuitive eating, but Evelyn Tribole, coauthor of Intuitive Eating, describes that "Intuitive Eating [is] a broader philosophy, which includes physical activity for the sake of feeling good, rejecting the dieting mentality, using nutrition information without judgment, and respecting your body, regardless of how you feel about its shape." Mindful eating involves an awareness of the process of eating without any judgment and could be an equally appropriate approach for someone who is not ready to track his or her dietary intake with flexible dieting.

For many of us, intuitive eating is incredibly challenging. This is why most of us end up overweight and a good portion of us end up with eating disorders. Nevertheless, if you are one of the lucky ones who can listen to your hunger cues, a general awareness of your eating experience and respect for your body and health might be what you need. Intuitive eating can also be a good approach for you if you do not have specific body composition or weight-related goals. Intuitive eating can also assist in improving long-term health or performance in activity and everyday life. It is also useful if you want to keep an eye on portion size without being strict enough to track dietary intake.

Tracking our intake is generally the most effective way to change our body weight. It is possible, however, to change your body weight without tracking your food intake. However, it is much more difficult because it requires a tremendous amount of self-control. Some of us restrict ourselves too much, but many of us eventually give in to the high-calorie, low-nutrient smorgasbord that is all around us.

To lose fat without tracking your intake, you must prioritize high-volume foods. As we know, ghrelin increases and leptin decreases as body weight decreases. Choose foods that are high in protein, fiber, water, and air to prevent unnecessary hunger. It is not that foods low in these components will prevent us from losing weight, but rather that they are not very satisfying and will leave us hungry and primed to go off-track. If we do not have a daily budget planned for ourselves, we must be committed to either saying no to "junk food" (high-calorie, high-fat, and/or high-sugar foods) or stopping after one or a few bites of these foods. It is also wise to keep in mind that fat is calorically dense, and we should consume high-fat foods in much smaller portions than many of us think. However, if you choose to follow a very low-carbohydrate diet, then you will need to follow a higher-fat diet.

If you do not want to track everything you eat forever but are willing to try it temporarily, flexible dieting can also be a great bridge into intuitive eating. Once you feel comfortable that you understand what your body needs to reach your goals, you can begin to estimate all portions instead of tracking numbers.

Remember that health is a state of balance, so if you can find that balance of getting enough but not too much of both nutrients and pleasure from your diet, then take an intuitive approach and forgo tracking. If you can reach your fitness goals without tracking, then do not worry about adding another layer of complexity to your life. However, if you find yourself taking an unhealthy extreme, restricting your body from nutrients, or stuffing yourself with food or negative thoughts, then tracking your intake, even for just a short period of time, can help you reach your goals. And even if you are reaching your goals with an intuitive approach but you want to see if you can fine-tune your nutrition to see even better results, then you might want to give flexible dieting a shot.

## Clean Eating

Clean eating involves eating a diet rich in whole foods. Whole foods are unprocessed or minimally processed and typically free from additives and other artificial ingredients. Despite the downfall of missing out on measuring exact portions, clean eating can generally help to ensure that you are getting adequate nutrients without overeating due to the nutrient content and satiating quality of whole foods. Like intuitive eating, clean eating can be a great approach if you are interested in improving long-term health or performance.

Clean eating is a dangerous game. A diet "rich in whole foods" can easily become a diet consisting only of whole foods. Once you start restricting yourself from certain foods, you begin to associate those foods with negative outcomes, and meals that could have been shared with loved ones become scary or "bad." If you have a history of disordered eating, then clean eating might not be your best bet.

It is still possible to overeat and create health issues by eating "clean" foods. We cannot cure modern illness by consuming only the foods that our hunter-gatherer ancestors ate. Our brains are wired to reward highly palatable foods. While it is more difficult to overeat foods that are high in fiber and protein, it is still possible. Many foods that our ancestors ate are much easier to overeat, like fatty meat, nuts, seeds, fruit, sweet potatoes, and honey. Anything that tastes good has a reward response in our brain, releasing dopamine and telling us to eat more of it. In addition, our level of physical activity does not match that of our ancestors. So much in our daily lives today is automatic and instantaneous. Most of us do not need to put in much manual labor to get things done.

A clean eating approach can also be difficult if you are trying to gain weight. Nutrient-dense, whole foods are often very filling due to their volume and fiber content. As one example, in the peak of my offseason from bodybuilding, desperate to fight my genetics and add mere ounces of muscle to my frame, I switched from salads and whole grains to bagels and cereal for two of my main carbohydrate sources.

On its own, clean eating is not the best way to reach body composition or weight goals, but you can easily layer some portion control on top to improve overall health and reach your bodyweight goals.

## Harm Reduction

Many people will tell you that if you want to start flexible dieting or take control of your diet in any way, you need to suck it up and go all in. I'm here to tell you that is not true. If you are only ready to take a small step, take it. There is no use staying at the starting line if you are ready to start the race. This type of gradual approach is often called a stepwise approach. Regarding harmful behaviors, this type of approach is often called harm reduction.

If your current diet is perpetuating negative thoughts or behaviors, an unhealthy body weight or body fat percentage, or other unhealthy outcomes, you can reduce the harm that you are doing by first pinpointing causes of the issues and then taking steps to reduce the harm. For example, if you are not ready to commit to tracking your intake, consider where the problems are coming from. What are the barriers to your success? Mindless snacking? Going off-track on the weekends? Restricting and binging?

Once you can pinpoint where the issues are coming from, focus on taking small steps to alleviate the negative impact. Reducing servings of sugary or fatty foods is an easy way to cut calories. Substituting them with a source of protein or fiber will help curb hunger. Imagine someone's typical day of eating is made up of 120 g fat, 50 g protein, and 300 g carbohydrates, and the person wants to "tone" up but does not want to track what he or she eats or exercise. The person can look for ways to cut out fat and carbohydrates and substitute some of those calories with protein and perhaps even begin resistance training once per week. This does not involve tracking anything. Once these habits are locked in, he or she can add in more new behaviors to further progress.

Life is a journey. To accomplish great things, we must take small steps. A successful diet is no different. Changes do not happen overnight. We have no choice but to take it one day at a time. Whether it is fitting in ten minutes of exercise today, allowing yourself to enjoy an occasional jelly bean instead of labeling it as "bad," or eliminating your lunchtime soda to cut back on overall calories, a small step is always better than no step.

With a harm reduction approach, you must still give 100% effort to a small step. If you find yourself only able to give 50% effort to your diet approach, then it might be time to see if you need to take a stepwise approach instead of jumping straight in. What small step are you ready to commit to 100%?

## Do What Works for You

We have discussed the principles necessary for a successful nutrition approach and the fact that these principles will vary depending on your specific goals. There are endless options that can help you accomplish and surpass your goals if you have a basic understanding of nutrition and your own situation and goals.

Even if you do not want to implement flexible dieting in your own life, aspects of flexible dieting can be applied to whichever approach you choose. Portion control is one of the fundamental components of flexible dieting that is a tried and true way to reach bodyweight goals. To reach body composition goals, you will need to incorporate your understanding of macronutrients into your meal planning.

If you do not want to be flexible in your approach at all, you can utilize your knowledge of nutrients to come up with a meal plan. Regardless of which approach works best for you, understanding what you are doing and why you are doing it is critical to your success. The media are plagued by marketing gimmicks and misleading information about nutrition. Creating your own base of knowledge about your own body is your best defense.

# 15
# BEWARE OF THE FADS AND GIMMICKS

The food industry is driven by sales. The fitness industry is driven by sales. The supplement industry is driven by sales. Watch out for sensationalized marketing techniques because the primary goal is always to get your money—not to improve your health. An endless number of approaches are taken in an attempt to sell you the next "best" thing.

You have probably come across advertisements for supplements or products that you "must buy." Notice that nothing in this book suggests that you need to buy a specific brand product. People will try to sell you products because it is their job, not because you need them.

To lose weight, you must burn more energy than you consume; to gain weight, you must consume more energy than you burn. To improve your body composition or your overall health, you must pay attention to the nutrient composition of your diet and your type and amount of physical activity. There is nothing that can take the place of a balanced diet and appropriate exercise, yet many companies claim to have secrets that can get us what we want without requiring us to work for them. Let's examine a few approaches to look out for.

## The "Quick Fix" Approach

The "quick fix" approach preys on our desire for immediate gratification. Why work for results later when you can have them now? These approaches advertise secrets that can unlock your potential and produce results much faster than traditional hard work and consistency.

Watch out for diets that tell you to target specific foods or supplements. Nutrition is a science, not magic. There is no single food or food group that you can add or eliminate to solve everything. There is no one workout program that will give you your dream physique in just a few weeks. There is not any pill or product that will do anything for you if you do not put the work in yourself.

Sometimes the media make us worry that we might have an allergy or an intolerance, or even worse that humans just are not meant to consume a specific food or food group. You may have heard somewhere that gluten or bread or dairy or sugar or grains or some other target food will make you sick or fat or cause other unwanted results. These claims serve as excuses for us to buy products that are free of these dangerous components. "Gluten-free" and "sugar-free" are two common labels to attract those of us wanting a quick fix by eliminating foods.

If you do not have an allergy, intolerance, or diagnosis, it is unnecessary to eliminate anything from your diet. Doing so is not a quick fix but a way to waste money. "You just need to do this one simple thing to solve all your problems." This approach is never the answer.

If you indeed have an allergy or intolerance that involves trouble metabolizing a food, it could lead to lower caloric intake overall from malabsorption. It would not make you fat.

Some quick fixes are effective. Extremely low-calorie diets will make you lose weight. You do not need to give anyone your money to unlock that secret. Quick fixes are seldom sustainable or healthy. Rapid weight loss is a great way to lose weight from muscle, water, and even bone.

To accomplish any goal, you must endure challenges. Change creates growth. If you are in a caloric deficit, you will feel like you are starving at times. As with anything else in life, it takes time and effort to be successful with your diet.

## The Confusion Approach

A great way to make people intrigued is to make something seem more complicated than it is. If "eat less; move more" cannot summarize a weight loss program, there is a red flag. You may have stumbled upon web pages about strategies to burn belly fat or improve digestion or build muscle that ask you to watch hour-long videos or read through several pages of text. The information is often intentionally confusing. You might be asked to subscribe to a long-term plan or to purchase one or more guides that will explain all the secrets of the product. You might be showered with information about supplements that you need to be taking.

If you ever feel inundated with information while browsing diets or products, keep in mind that confusion is a marketing tactic. Providing you with confusing, excessive information prevents you from being able to compare what they are offering with what others are offering.

As we have mentioned before, some nutrition approaches claim that they have an exclusive, secret answer. For instance, foods should only be eaten in certain combinations to lose weight. There is no "wrong" combination of foods that will produce poor results. There are no secrets to success when it comes to dieting. Using many words to describe unusual, unproven approaches do not validate them. Anyone can claim to have discovered a new technique that is better than the rest, one that requires you to spend hours of your time learning about them or to just "trust them" because they use a lot of words.

Arguments for approaches that claim that "there's just so much that we don't know" should make you think twice. We know quite a lot. We know about macronutrients and micronutrients and nonnutritive compounds. We know about energy balance. We have all the tools we need to reach our fitness goals. There are no secrets. If someone is telling you otherwise, you need to  step back and find a science-based, sustainable approach.

## The Endorsement Approach

If you attach a famous face to anything, people will probably like that thing more. This is common with weight loss and athletic performance products. However, just because someone poses with, gives a speech about, or even writes a book about a product does not mean that the product is what gave the person results. More importantly, it does not mean that using this product is the best approach for you. Social media makes it easy to make it seem like celebrities are endorsing products that they are not. Fake tweets and videos taken out of context are examples of this.

An endorsement does not have to come from a traditional celebrity for it to be effective. Other examples include educated individuals. An MD, PhD, RD, or other degree or certification after a name gain attention. It makes sense; we think someone who has experience in the field can be considered an expert or at least relied on for advice. However, social media gurus with large followings and strong self-marketing are also often looked up to as experts. While successfully marketing your personal brand to attract thousands or even millions of followers on social media earns you a certain type of fame, social media success by itself does not give you credibility.

Just because something is publicized and endorsed does not mean it is true, safe, or effective. Do not be fooled by a friendly face or a degree advertising a diet or product. Would you still be interested in the same diet or product without the endorsement? Can you verify that the diet or product is built on sound, scientific principles, or does it simply fall into one or more of these other approaches?

## The Intimate Approach

"The customer is the product." With the intimate approach, we are often sold an experience rather than a product. Emotion often has a greater influence than content on our purchasing patterns. Brand name products are more expensive than their generic counterparts, but many of us prefer to buy brand name products because of the mental image of the brand we carry in our minds from seeing advertisements for the brand.

Something does not have to be rational or correct for us to buy it. The IPA databank of successful advertising campaigns suggests that campaigns with only emotional content may be about twice as successful as those with only rational content.

Some products tease you with a sense of belonging: "Join thousands of others just like you!" Maybe it is the cool, trendy thing to do. Even new products or programs try to grant you a sense of belonging; "be one of the first to try our new program!" You can be a leader. "You'll regret it if you don't!"

In diet advertising, even negative emotions like fear and guilt are common and effective: "Don't let this happen to you!" "Don't keep doing this to yourself!" A New York Times viral content study showed that even some negative emotions, like anger and anxiety, are associated with virality of content.

When you are faced with advertisements that promise to make you happy and feel great, remember that self-acceptance is a journey. There is no time in the future when you will feel entirely confident every second of every day. Everyone has ups and downs.

Sometimes the intimate approach targets specific audiences rather than specific emotions. We are all people. Nutrition should be personalized, not simply divided into different programs based on a single variable. Be wary of ads that act like men and women are two different species, for example.

## The Restrictive Approach

If you want results, you must be extreme, right? It makes sense to assume that if we cut out all processed foods and added sugar, we will have the best possible results. However, we often forget that restriction is a very dangerous path. Each food that we eliminate might just increase our risk of getting inadequate nutrients or worsening our mental health. Additionally, a restrictive approach is a great way to get you to spend your money learning about the approach and all its cult-like following and by buying specialty products, cookbooks, programs, and more.

Once I told a health professional about how much weight I unintentionally lost when I followed a raw vegan diet and consumed up to fourteen bananas in one day. She told me, "That's because it didn't stick." Some people think that fruit and vegetables have some magic component that other sources of carbohydrates lack. There is no magic in food. Fruit "sticks" just fine. I lost weight because I was not consuming enough calories. The high fiber and water content was so satiating that I was not consuming as many calories as I should have been.

What I do not know, however, is exactly how many total calories and how many grams of fiber I was consuming. In fact, she may have been onto something; most fiber passes through the digestive tract undigested, so a portion of the food I was consuming was not being digested and absorbed. My bowel movements can confirm this. As part of a balanced diet, fruit and vegetables are healthy. But if you are only eating fruit and vegetables, as I once was when I neared the end of my time as a raw vegan, your diet can become very problematic. You can replace "fruit and vegetables" with just about any food, and the same will be true. Moderation is safe; restriction can be dangerous.

One of the main problems with very restrictive diets that require very low or no intake of several types of food is that they inevitably lead to excess intake of certain nutrients and inadequate intake of others. On my raw vegan diet, for example, I was not getting enough protein, fat, B vitamins, creatine, carnosine, vitamin D, and other key nutrients. A balanced diet is high in variety. A variety of foods means a variety of nutrients. If you consume a diet with high variety, one specific food will not make a difference. However, if your diet is low in variety, then one specific food can in fact make a noticeable difference in your health.

Diets that allow you to eat an unlimited amount of certain foods and eliminate others are bogus. Food has calories, so an unlimited number of calories will tip your energy balance in the wrong direction. Moreover, it will be boring and difficult to follow, and you may end up with too much of certain nutrients and too little of others.

Work smarter, not harder.

## The Keyword Approach

The title of an article written by Morgan McCloy for NPR in January 2016 reads, "Diet Foods Are Tanking. So the Diet Industry Is Now Selling 'Health.'" Products are now sold with attractive labels slapped on to attract health-conscious consumers; organic, non-GMO, diet, high protein, gluten-free, and detox are just some of these labels. Simply adding a label to something does not make it a better option than something else without a good marketing strategy behind it. Spinach is all natural, but you probably will not find a "natural" keyword written across its packaging (if it has any).

We may grab products with "healthy" labels without even knowing what they mean. The FDA does not have a definition for natural. USDA standards for "organic" vary depending on whether it is produce, meat, or a processed, multi-ingredient food. "Made with organic ingredients" means at least 70% of the ingredients are organically produced. If a product is labeled "organic," but not "USDA organic," it could mean anything. There are so many keywords that are used to make products and entire dietary approached more appealing for health-conscious consumers.

"Detox" is one keyword that can unnecessarily negatively impact your wallet and your health. Detox diets often claim that the body accumulates toxins and waste that can be removed by eating specific foods or drinking specific beverages and eliminating others entirely. However, our bodies naturally detoxify via the liver and kidneys, and the Academy of Nutrition and Dietetics (AND) recommends that we help your body detoxify by consuming a balanced diet and drinking enough water, not by consuming high quantities of certain foods or beverages and avoiding others.

A detox diet is just one of the many diets that take advantage of keywords. Caveman, paleo, vegan, low-carb, low-fat: the list goes on. There is no need to restrict unless you personally have an issue with certain foods. These diets can be harmful if they are not balanced enough to provide adequate nutrients. A sustainable, balanced approach is ideal. The dose makes the poison. Any negative effect from a single food comes from overconsumption of that food, not from consuming the food at all.

## Look Past the Marketing

Good advertising does not make a good product. When a diet or product catches your eye, take some time to understand the way it works and to make sure its claims are backed by science. Do not be afraid to do research yourself. What scientific studies were published on the topic? How can you apply these findings to your practice?

When it comes to diet, critical thinking can help you save your health and money. Always use common sense, and remember that reward comes from work. Aside from genetics, there is no luck involved in reaching nutrition goals. Hard work, consistency, and patience are key ingredients for success. Tricks and tips to lose weight fast that do not involve increasing expenditure or decreasing intake are bogus.

Moreover, just because a product description references a scientific study does not mean that the product does what it claims. Citing one study is often a red flag because studies on the same topic produce conflicting data all the time. We need to look at the bigger picture. Who funded the study? What was the study design? The randomized trial is the gold standard, and even those have faults. What was the sample size? What methods were used? Have any other studies found similar or conflicting results? Have any reviews been published? We need to be critical thinkers when we make decisions that can positively or negatively impact our health. Do not fall for the latest trend or keyword.

Marketing is designed to target you, but it does not know you. Only you can identify your own problem areas and figure out where you can improve. Get away from analyzing specific foods and look at your overall dietary pattern. As much as we like shortcuts, results can only be produced by a lot of hard work, consistency, and patience.

# 16
# CONCLUSION

There are people in this world who will tell you that you need to change your lifestyle to reach your goals, that you need to sacrifice all of life's pleasures to lose weight, that you need to fuel your body with only unprocessed foods to be healthy. But none of this is true. In fact, you can do any or all of these things and still be unsuccessful. If you take away nothing else from this book, at least remember these two phrases: the dose makes the poison, and the best diet is the one you can stick to.

"The dose makes the poison." No single food can do you harm if it is part of a balanced diet. How do we ensure a balanced diet? Follow correct calories and macronutrients to reach your goals, aim for variety, eat more unsaturated than saturated fats, get most calories from plants, use more high-quality protein sources than supplements, and eat more low or medium GI carbs than high GI carbs (especially when added sugars are involved). The result is a balanced diet with room for flexibility.

"The best diet is the one you can stick to." Nutrition is an integral part of health. Regardless of your fitness goals, your diet should aid both your physical and mental health. Remember what really matters to you. There are more important things in life than the foods you eat. Don't compromise yourself on account of a diet. From ice cream with the kids to a steak dinner with your significant other, you can still stay on track if you plan around these special occasions.

Sure, in an ideal world, we would each have farms, cook all our food, and get most of our calories from plants, but no such utopia exists. Instead we create the boundaries of our diet and fill it in with whatever fits our lifestyle. With flexible dieting, we compromise neither our goals nor our lifestyle because both must work together. We do not have to create a picture-perfect, farm-to-table world where we only consume fresh, whole foods. We also do not have to eliminate anything because it is "bad." We just need to understand how much of each nutrient we need to reach our goals and then consume a balanced diet to get close to these values.

You can in fact eat whatever you want and reach your goals. You just need to eat what you want in appropriate amounts. Flexible dieting has the potential to be so effortless that no one around you ever knows if you are dieting, maintaining, or gaining weight. In fact, people usually guess incorrectly when they ask me what my current goal is.

Flexible dieting saved my sanity if not my life. In 2012, I moved back to the United States from France and promptly started a raw vegan diet. I thought I was pursuing health, but I was pursuing purity, which is one of the dumbest things you can do with your diet. Nothing is pure. I kept eliminating more and more foods until I was eating only fruit and vegetables, and finally I felt guilty for even eating bananas. "Who am I to take this banana from the earth?" I thought. I saw myself as below bananas on the food chain, and that is when I knew I had a problem. Somehow the BMI of 15, hair loss, fatigue, skin problems, lack of desire to socialize or exist beyond schoolwork, and utter obsession with my "health" were not effective enough red flags for me.

When I finally realized the danger of my approach, I began a journey to recover my mental and physical health. I tried standard vegan, pescatarian, ketogenic, and "clean eating" diets as I tried to improve my health. But with all these diets, I had to follow an elimination mentality. I had to agree to live the rest of my life without touching many if not most meal options ever again. More importantly, I had to agree to do this for no good reason. I do not have significant food allergies or intolerances, and I do not have any major health diagnoses. Moreover, I have access to sustainably sourced, excellent-quality food from all food groups. I also love bananas and spinach and peanut butter and salmon and tofu and nachos and ice cream and homemade cookies, and there is a place for each of these foods in my diet and my life. None of my favorite foods is "bad" for me because all my favorite foods are foods. Just like me, you need calories to survive, and you deserve to enjoy the act of eating.

The problem with the elimination mentality is that it wrongly defines what it means to be healthy. Being healthy is not an extreme situation that exists on the far end of a spectrum. Rather, being healthy is a stable equilibrium that can be achieved by finding our own personal version of balance. Until I started studying nutrition, I thought health was an extreme. For years, I pursued that extreme until I finally noticed there were negative effects on both my physical and mental health.

My first experience with true healthy eating wasn't until I moved to Paris, France, when I was eighteen years old. At the time, I thought, "Wow, these people are not as healthy as everyone thinks." Years later, I realized that the stereotype was right all along. Many French families serve salad as a starter or a side; meat, vegetables, and starches as the main course; and cheese, bread, and dessert for the final course. Special occasions might require aperitifs (appetizers), where people nibble on meat, cheese, crackers and sip on an alcoholic beverage. For dessert, I was usually offered a small serving of yogurt, fruit, or a more typical American dessert, like ice cream, flan, or a brownie. The portions for everything are small by American standards. When you order a soda at a restaurant, you might get a small glass bottle that looks to be 8 fl oz or so. Alcohol is common at meals, but usually only a glass or two. In traditional French eating, excess does not have a place. But neither does restriction. Children are exposed to a wide range of foods at a young age instead of monster servings of high-fat, high-sugar, high-sodium concoctions from the pantry section of the grocery store.

There is this idea out there that you can either live a life of pleasure or a life of health, but you cannot have both. Some people think, "Well, I could never commit to that. I don't have that kind of willpower." So, they don't even try. Meanwhile, a harm reduction approach would be much more effective. The big secret not just to optimizing your health but to succeeding in whatever you do is to find your balance. We each have twenty four hours each day that we choose to spend however we want. Some of us work twelve hours a day and feel good about it; others value time with family or friends instead. One is no better than the other.

Here is the question that you must ask yourself to find out if you are ready to diet: are you ready to sacrifice your love of eating for your goals? Many people complain that they can never lose weight because they are simply not ready to give up the freedom and pleasure of eating whatever, whenever. But you do not need to be prepared to sacrifice your love of eating to start flexible dieting. You just need to be aware of the nutritional value of what you are eating so you can eat portions that fit within your calorie and nutrient goals.

The next time you are presented with an opportunity to eat a slice of birthday cake, you do not have to say no. You just have to decide what size slice you are willing to fit into your daily budget or if you would rather opt for a lower-calorie treat.

A typical complimentary boxed lunch at work or school events includes a deli meat sandwich, chips, a cookie, and an apple. There are two main reactions to this kind of free lunch: (1) eat what you like without thinking twice and maybe even grab an extra of one or more elements, or (2) avoid one or more elements that you "shouldn't" be eating. The first is driven by personal desires, and the second is driven by personal pressure.

Deli meat, bread, chips, cookies, and even apples have each been labeled "bad." Preservatives, gluten, processed foods, high-fat, high-sodium, added sugars, and fruit have all been targeted at some point.

A pressure-based approach can involve a multitude of pressures, but the one that we need to be listening to is logic. When we are faced with a decision about what to eat, like when we are given a free boxed lunch, a logical approach is one that involves math. We can subtract the approximate grams of fat, carbohydrates, and protein from our daily target guidelines. What fits in your daily budget depends on your metabolic rate and goals.

By contrast, a desire-based approach involves choosing to eat what we want. What are you hungry for? What do you like?

Successfully reaching our nutrition and health goals requires marrying both the pressure-based and the desire-based approaches. Tracking your intake is just one tool in the toolbox. Remember that successful flexible dieting involves an appreciation of yourself and the fact that every day is new and different.

Most of us will not be able to have every meal look like the USDA MyPlate. Most of us do not eat only whole, unprocessed foods. The aisles of the grocery store are filled with items that have long lists of ingredients. When we look at the numbers that represent the nutrients, we can easily see that it is okay if our meals are not perfect representations of the MyPlate. While some people do succeed at having all or most meals resemble this kind of template, most of us do not live a lifestyle that supports this or even have the motivation to follow through with such extreme behavior. (Today in America, eating whole foods for every single meal is extreme behavior.) But most of us can learn to understand the nutrient content of foods and budget for the things that we need and the things we want. We already do it with money.

Some people will tell you that you need to change your lifestyle to change your diet. They will tell you that you need to see food as fuel, that it takes x number of days to build a habit. It's like saying, "You just need to change your entire way of thinking. You just need to change yourself." It's absurd, really. You don't have to change yourself to become healthy. It is not a black-and-white issue.

For people who already drink alcohol, the recommendation is moderate consumption. For people who already consume artificial sweeteners, the recommendation is moderate consumption. Why don't we treat food the same way? Many of us consume highly palatable and/or processed foods as part of our normal dietary intake. We do not need to recommend that someone who does not eat any fast food should eat it, but for someone who already does eat fast food, recommending a moderate consumption, such as one to two servings per week, could be beneficial. There is a misleading division between those of us who "eat healthy" and those of us who "don't eat healthy." Let's bridge the gap.

## End the Obsession

The danger of IIFYM is thinking that hitting your macronutrient intake goals is enough. While most food weight is made up of macronutrients and water, there are other compounds found in food that are critical to overall health. However, consuming a balanced diet does not mean we should obsess about specific foods or nutrients. Which foods are healthy? Which ones should I avoid? Which foods will help me lose weight? Which foods will make me gain weight? Which vitamins do I need to take?

Many people latch on to any claim about "good" or "bad" foods, but they miss the bigger picture and never reach their goals. Just because salmon is nutrient-dense does not mean you should eat it every single night. If the rest of your diet is high in fat, then the salmon might be pushing you over the edge into a diet that has too much fat. If you are already eating in a caloric surplus, then the salmon is only going to add more calories. Just because you avoid sugar, gluten, or anything else that you heard rumors about does not necessarily mean you will be any healthier.

Perfect is the enemy of good. If we think that we are unable to achieve a perfect diet, sometimes we avoid doing what is good. And sometimes when we try to achieve a perfect diet, we may realize that we are pursuing a diet that is not only unsustainable but also potentially detrimental. It is only when you understand the quantity of food that you need to be eating that you should start examining the quality of the food. Once you know how many daily calories you need, you can look at macronutrients and then micronutrients, and lastly you can figure out which foods best fill these requirements.

The overall composition of your diet is and always will be what matters most. No single food or nutrient can change the fact that energy balance is best represented by an equation. On one side of the equation lies all the energy you consume from food. On the other side lies all the energy your body burns from activities. It truly does not matter how many "healthy" foods you consume if the "wrong" side of the equation is greater.

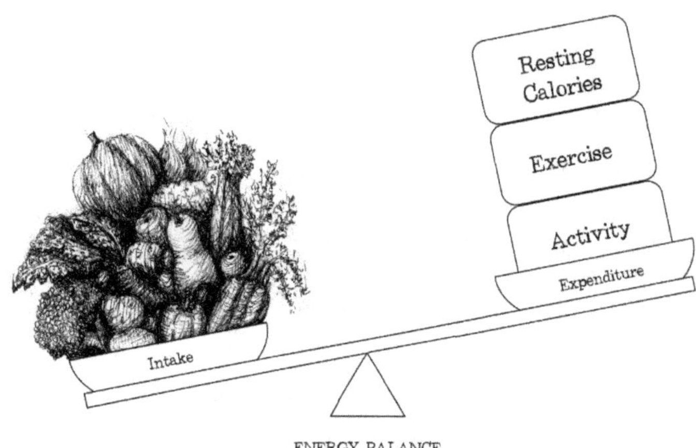



ENERGY BALANCE

If you know the scale is tipped in the right direction, and you still are not seeing progress, it does not mean that it is time to start blaming specific foods. Rather, you might need to look at your nutrient intake. Carbohydrates, protein, and fat each have different effects on the body. If your calorie intake is appropriate but your macronutrient intake is not conducive to your goals, you simply will not make the progress you are hoping for. For example, if you restrict calories because you want to lose fat and look toned, and you end up losing weight but looking flabby rather than toned, then you might need to increase your protein intake and strength training and reduce carbohydrate or fat intake. Once macronutrient composition is set, food choice becomes much easier because we know not to spend our calorie budget on chips and cookies.

If you ever find yourself obsessing over which foods are best to eat, zoom out and look at the bigger picture. Psychology plays a critical yet often forgotten role in nutrition. A perfect diet will not give you perfect health, but a balanced diet can help you improve physical and mental health.

The two simple actions of being mindful about what you put into your body and what you do with your body are overcomplicated by the media, the public, and even professionals. The best advice anyone can ever give you is to take care of yourself as if it were the most important thing in the world—because you are. Enjoy the journey!

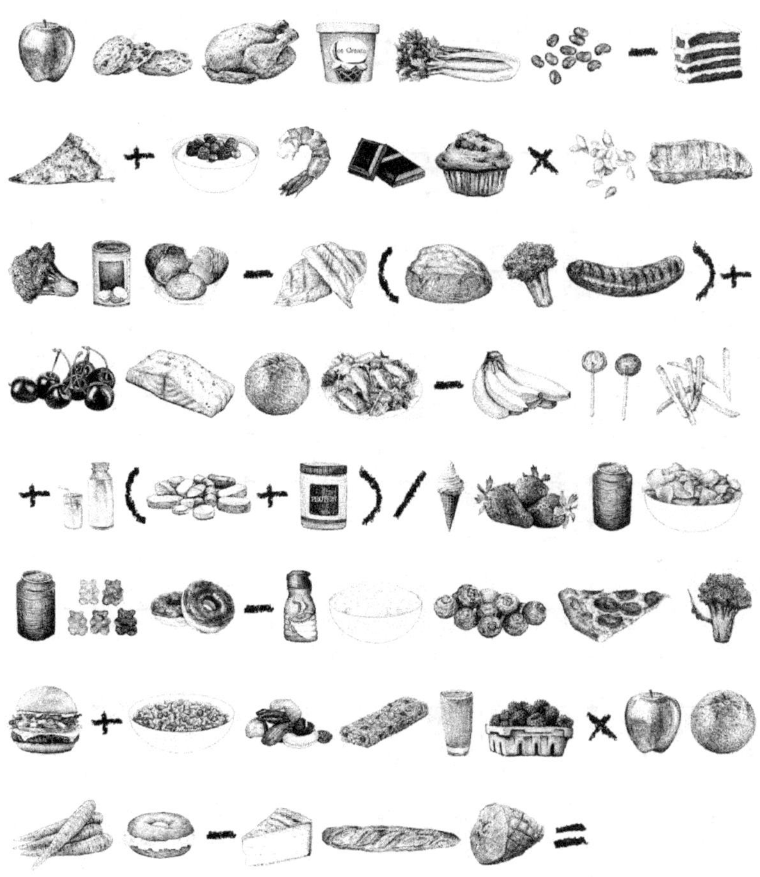

# The Dose Makes The Poison

# 17
# MACRO-FRIENDLY MEAL OPTIONS

| Restaurant | Meal | Fat (g) | Carb (g) | Prot (g) |
|---|---|---|---|---|
| Applebee's | Chili | 18 | 14 | 27 |
| Applebee's | Grilled Chicken Wonton Tacos | 13 | 35 | 27 |
| Applebee's | 8 oz USDA Top Sirloin | 10 | 2 | 45 |
| Applebee's | Steamed Broccoli | 8 | 6 | 3 |
| Applebee's | Pepper-Encrusted Sirloin & Whole Grains | 14 | 48 | 32 |
| Applebee's | Thai Shrimp Salad | 19 | 32 | 23 |
| Applebee's | Kids' Chicken Griller | 4 | 1 | 38 |
| Burger King | Tendergrill Chicken Sandwich (No Mayo) | 6 | 35 | 32 |
| Burger King | Chicken Nugget 4pc | 11 | 11 | 8 |
| Burger King | Grilled Chicken Salad with Tendergrill | 14 | 16 | 36 |
| California Pizza Kitchen | Bianco Flatbread | 15 | 38 | 18 |
| California Pizza Kitchen | Shaved Mushroom & Spinach Flatbread | 18 | 40 | 18 |
| California Pizza Kitchen | 1/2 Lunch Size Pizza | 12 | 45 | 15 |
| California Pizza Kitchen | Shrimp Scampi Zucchini | 24 | 30 | 27 |
| California Pizza Kitchen | Kids' Chicken Breast | 6 | 9 | 39 |
| Carrabba's | Grilled Asparagus with Prosciutto | 6 | 5 | 18 |
| Carrabba's | Italian Lettuce Wraps | 10 | 11 | 18 |
| Carrabba's | Chicken Soup (Bowl) | 5 | 20 | 16 |
| Carrabba's | Tuscan Grilled Chicken | 7 | <1 | 52 |
| Carrabba's | Plain Steamed Broccoli | 0 | 8 | 3 |
| Carrabba's | Plain Steamed Asparagus | 0 | 4 | 2 |
| Carrabba's | Plain Steamed Green Beans | 0 | 6 | 2 |
| Carrabba's | Chicken Parmesan Sandwich (Half) | 9 | 33 | 22 |
| Chick-fil-A | Grilled Chicken Sandwich | 6 | 36 | 29 |
| Chick-fil-A | Nuggets | 12 | 9 | 28 |

| Restaurant | Meal | Fat (g) | Carb (g) | Prot (g) |
|---|---|---|---|---|
| Chick-fil-A | Grilled Nuggets | 3.5 | 2 | 25 |
| Chick-fil-A | Egg White Grill | 7 | 31 | 25 |
| Chick-fil-A | Grilled Market Salad | 6 | 15 | 25 |
| Chick-fil-A | Fruit Cup | 0 | 12 | 0 |
| Chick-fil-A | Side Salad | 4.5 | 6 | 5 |
| Chili's | Seared Shrimp - Full Order | 3 | 2 | 13 |
| Chili's | Steamed Broccoli | 0 | 8 | 3 |
| Chili's | Asparagus & Garlic Roasted Tomatoes | 1.5 | 12 | 4 |
| Chili's | 6 oz Sirloin w/ Grilled Avocado | 20 | 23 | 39 |
| Chili's | Mango-Chile Tilapia | 19 | 55 | 38 |
| Chili's | Margarita Grilled Chicken | 14 | 64 | 51 |
| Chili's | House Salad (No Dressing) | 3.5 | 8 | 3 |
| Denny's | BYOGS: 2 Turkey Bacon, 2 Egg White | 10 | 4 | 36 |
| Denny's | BYOGS: Turkey Bacon, Plain English Muffin, 2 Egg White | 7 | 32 | 34 |
| Denny's | BYOGS: Turkey Bacon, Fruit, 2 Egg White | 6 | 21 | 31 |
| Denny's | Grilled Seasoned Chicken Breast | 6 | 1 | 35 |
| Denny's | Cranberry Apple Chicken Salad | 9 | 36 | 36 |
| IHOP | Simple & Fit Veggie Omelette (No Fruit) | 10 | 27 | 27 |
| IHOP | Simple & Fit Two-Egg Breakfast | 8 | 48 | 25 |
| McDonald's | Bacon Ranch Grilled Chicken Salad | 14 | 9 | 42 |
| McDonald's | Southwest Grilled Chicken Salad | 12 | 27 | 37 |
| McDonald's | Egg White Delight | 8 | 29 | 16 |
| McDonald's | Apple Slices | 0 | 4 | 0 |
| McDonald's | Side Salad | 0 | 3 | 1 |
| McDonald's | Artisan Grilled Chicken Sandwich | 7 | 44 | 37 |
| McDonald's | Chicken McNuggets 4pc | 11 | 11 | 10 |
| McDonald's | Vanilla Ice Cream Cone | 5 | 23 | 5 |
| The Melting Pot | Spinach Mushroom Salad (No Dressing) | 1 | 4 | 2 |
| The Melting Pot | Chicken (Coq au Vin, Court Bouillon, Mojo) | 3 | 1 | 53 |

| Restaurant | Meal | Fat (g) | Carb (g) | Prot (g) |
|---|---|---|---|---|
| The Melting Pot | Lobster Tail (Coq au Vin, Court Bouillon, Mojo) | 0 | 6 | 37 |
| The Melting Pot | Angus Sirloin (Coq au Vin, Court Bouillon, Mojo) | 10 | 9 | 51 |
| The Melting Pot | Mahi Mahi (Coq au Vin, Court Bouillon, Mojo) | 2 | 1 | 40 |
| The Melting Pot | Vegetable Medley | 0 | 13 | 3 |
| The Melting Pot | Citrus Soy Sauce | 0 | 4 | 1 |
| The Melting Pot | Green Goddess Sauce | 3 | 1 | 1 |
| The Melting Pot | Teriyaki Glaze | 0 | 3 | 0 |
| Olive Garden | House Salad (No Dressing) | 2 | 10 | 2 |
| Olive Garden | House Salad (Low-Fat Dressing) | 4 | 12 | 2 |
| Olive Garden | Herb-Grilled Salmon | 28 | 8 | 43 |
| Olive Garden | Tilapia Piccata | 22 | 11 | 46 |
| Olive Garden | Steamed Broccoli | 0 | 4 | 2 |
| Olive Garden | Kids' Spaghetti w/ Grilled Chicken (No Sauce) | 5 | 33 | 34 |
| Olive Garden | Mini Strawberry & White Chocolate Cake | 11 | 23 | 1 |
| Olive Garden | Breadstick (with garlic topping) | 2.5 | 25 | 4 |
| Outback Steakhouse | Sesame Salad with Ahi Tuna | 8 | 15 | 33 |
| Outback Steakhouse | 6 oz Sirloin | 13 | 0 | 37 |
| Outback Steakhouse | 6 oz Victoria's Filet Mignon | 9 | 0 | 36 |
| Outback Steakhouse | Simply Grilled Mahi | 3.5 | 1 | 47 |
| Outback Steakhouse | Grilled Chicken on the Barbie | 3.5 | 11 | 57 |
| Outback Steakhouse | Grilled Asparagus | 4 | 4 | 2 |
| Outback Steakhouse | Seasonal Mixed Veggies | 9 | 15 | 4 |
| Outback Steakhouse | Steamed Broccoli | 9 | 12 | 5 |
| Outback Steakhouse | Sauteed Mushrooms | 6 | 10 | 7 |
| Panda Express | Broccoli Beef | 7 | 13 | 9 |
| Panda Express | Hot Szechuan Tofu | 8 | 10 | 6 |

| Restaurant | Meal | Fat (g) | Carb (g) | Prot (g) |
|---|---|---|---|---|
| Panda Express | Mushroom Chicken | 9 | 11 | 12 |
| Panda Express | String Bean Chicken Breast | 9 | 13 | 14 |
| Panda Express | Five Flavor Shrimp | 11 | 14 | 14 |
| Panda Express | Steamed Ginger Fish | 12 | 8 | 15 |
| Panera Bread | Low-Fat Chicken Noodle Soup (Cup) | 3 | 13 | 10 |
| Panera Bread | Thai Garden Chicken Wonton Bowl | 6 | 37 | 23 |
| Panera Bread | Strawberry & Poppyseed Chicken Salad | 13 | 33 | 29 |
| Pei Wei Asian Diner | Hot & Sour Soup (Bowl) | 6 | 15 | 12 |
| Pei Wei Asian Diner | Thai Basil Small with Chicken | 19 | 28 | 24 |
| Pei Wei Asian Diner | Korean Spicy Small with Chicken | 18 | 25 | 23 |
| Pei Wei Asian Diner | Thai Dynamite Small with Chicken (Steamed) | 18 | 25 | 26 |
| Pei Wei Asian Diner | Lettuce Cup (substitute for rice) | 0 | 6 | 2 |
| Pei Wei Asian Diner | Fortune Cookie | 0 | 5 | 0 |
| P. F. Chang's China Bistro | Handmade Shrimp Dumplings Steamed (4) | 2.5 | 21 | 19 |
| P. F. Chang's China Bistro | Wonton Soup Cup | 3 | 11 | 10 |
| P. F. Chang's China Bistro | Buddha's Feast Steamed | 4 | 32 | 26 |
| P. F. Chang's China Bistro | GF Ginger Chicken with Broccoli | 14 | 47 | 63 |
| Red Lobster | Signature Shrimp Cocktail | 0 | 11 | 21 |
| Red Lobster | Live Maine Lobster - Stuffed | 10 | 21 | 65 |
| Red Lobster | Broiled Flounder Dinner | 11 | 0 | 70 |
| Red Lobster | Fresh Broccoli | 0 | 8 | 39 |
| Red Lobster | Lighthouse Rock Lobster Tail | 14 | 35 | 45 |
| Red Lobster | Lighthouse Wood-Grilled Peppercorn Sirloin and Shrimp | 18 | 36 | 54 |
| Red Robin | Ensenada Chicken Platter | 18 | 27 | 61 |
| Red Robin | Ensenada Chicken Platter (One Chicken Breast) | 11 | 19 | 32 |
| Red Robin | Simply Grilled Chicken Salad | 8 | 25 | 37 |
| Ruby Tuesday | Fit & Trim Hickory Bourbon Chicken | 6 | 60 | 31 |
| Ruby Tuesday | Fit & Trim Petite Sirloin (6 oz) | 17 | 43 | 37 |

| Restaurant | Meal | Fat (g) | Carb (g) | Prot (g) |
|---|---|---|---|---|
| Ruby Tuesday | Fit & Trim Top Sirloin (8 oz) | 23 | 44 | 53 |
| Ruby Tuesday | Blackened Tilapia | 6 | 1 | 31 |
| Ruby Tuesday | New Orleans Seafood | 15 | 3 | 44 |
| Ruby Tuesday | 2 Shrimp Skewers | 6 | 0 | 12 |
| Ruby Tuesday | Hickory Bourbon Chicken | 5 | 18 | 26 |
| Ruby Tuesday | Chicken Bella | 16 | 8 | 36 |
| Ruby Tuesday | Petite Sirloin (6 oz) | 17 | 1 | 32 |
| Ruby Tuesday | Top Sirloin (8 oz) | 22 | 2 | 50 |
| Ruby Tuesday | Fresh Steamed Broccoli | 2 | 5 | 3 |
| Ruby Tuesday | Fresh Green Beans | 4 | 5 | 1 |
| Ruby Tuesday | Fresh Grilled Zucchini | 0 | 2 | 1 |
| Ruby Tuesday | Fresh Grilled Asparagus | 2 | 7 | 3 |
| Smoothie King | 20 oz Banana Gladiator Smoothie | 0 | 37 | 45 |
| Starbucks | Reduced-Fat Turkey Bacon & Cage Free Egg White Breakfast Sandwich | 6 | 28 | 16 |
| Starbucks | Sous Vide Egg Bites: Egg White & Red Pepper | 7 | 13 | 13 |
| Starbucks | Spinach, Feta & Cage Free Egg White Breakfast Wrap | 10 | 33 | 19 |
| Steak 'n Shake | Grilled Chicken Salad | 10 | 30 | 26 |
| Steak 'n Shake | Cottage Cheese w/ Pineapple Ring | 6 | 10 | 14 |
| Steak 'n Shake | Turkey Club Sandwich | 16 | 45 | 24 |
| Steak 'n Shake | 2 Eggs and 2 Slices of Bacon | 19 | 2 | 20 |
| Subway | Carved Turkey Salad | 3.5 | 12 | 20 |
| Subway | Oven Roasted Chicken Salad | 2.5 | 11 | 19 |
| Taco Bell | Shredded Chicken Mini Quesadilla | 8 | 15 | 12 |
| Taco Bell | Fresco Soft Taco - Shredded Chicken | 3.5 | 16 | 10 |
| Taco Bell | Fresco Soft Taco - Steak | 4 | 17 | 10 |
| Taco Bell | Cheese Roll-Up | 9 | 15 | 9 |
| Taco Bell | Crunchy Taco | 9 | 13 | 8 |

| Restaurant | Meal | Fat (g) | Carb (g) | Prot (g) |
|---|---|---|---|---|
| Wendy's | Grilled Chicken Sandwich | 8 | 38 | 35 |
| Wendy's | Grilled Chicken Wrap | 11 | 24 | 20 |
| Wendy's | Crispy Chicken Nuggets | 13 | 10 | 10 |
| Wendy's | Power Mediterranean Chicken Salad, Half | 9 | 22 | 20 |

# 18
# ABOUT THE AUTHORS

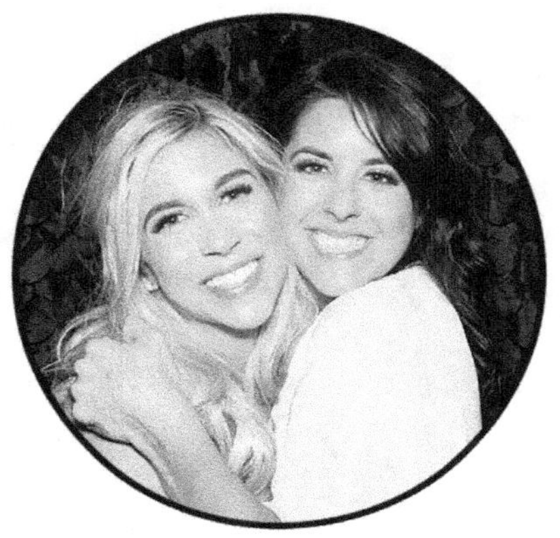

## The Author

Acadia Buro has an MS in Human Nutrition from Columbia University and is pursuing a PhD in Public Health at the University of South Florida. Her current research is in nutrition in children with autism spectrum disorder and low-income families. She has years of experience working in obesity nutrition research and is a certified nutrition coach and personal trainer. She has been coaching and mentoring clients since 2013. For more on Acadia visit: www.acadiafit.com

## The Illustrator

Hannah Merchant earned a BFA in Woodworking and Furniture Design with a minor in Public Engagement from the Maine College of Art in 2013. She has designed and built community projects in coastal Maine ranging from creating a tricycle-powered mobile farmstand, to sign building, to book compiling and design, and illustration. She currently lives along the coast of Maine where she is building a self-sufficient, off-the-grid home and homestead. She is passionate about connecting people to their community, the land through working with their hands, and the source of their food. For more on Hannah visit: www.dugnadfarm.com